Slimming World's
world of
flavours

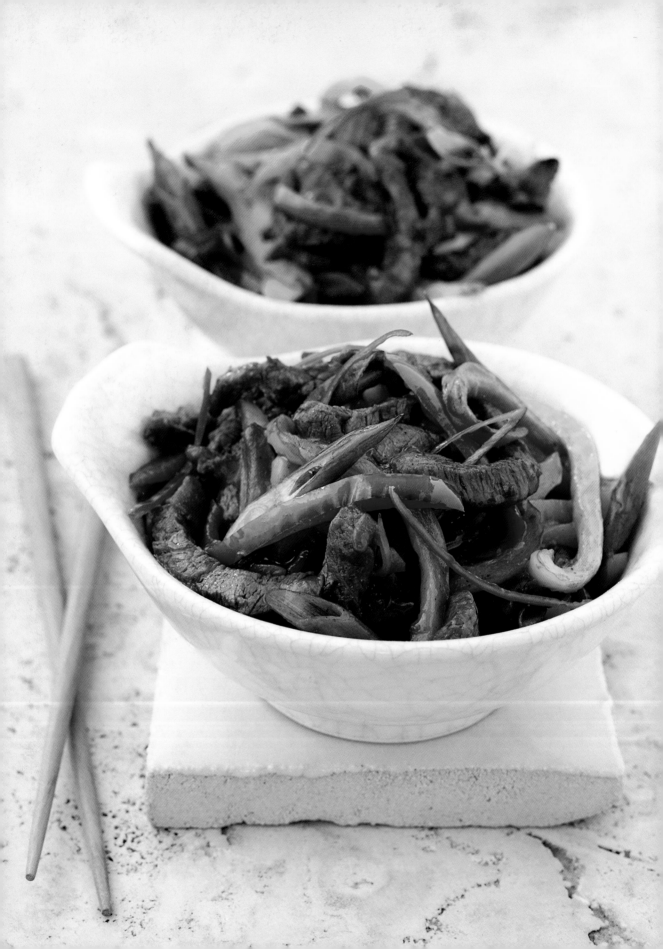

Slimming World's

world of

flavours

over 120 fresh, healthy and
delicious recipes from around the world

EBURY
PRESS

Cookery notes

- Both metric and imperial measures are given for the recipes. Choose one set of measures to follow as they are not interchangeable.

- All spoon measures are level:
  1 tsp = 5ml,
  1 tbsp = 15ml spoon.

- (V) Suitable for vegetarians.

- ✳ Suitable for freezing.

- Ovens should be preheated to the specified temperature. Grills should also be preheated.

- Use large eggs unless otherwise specified.

- Note that some of the recipes contain lightly cooked eggs. Avoid serving these to anyone who is pregnant or in a vulnerable health group, as there is a small risk of salmonella infection.

- All fruit and vegetables should be washed before use.

- Always use fresh herbs unless dried herbs are suggested in the recipe.

- Use freshly ground black pepper and sea salt unless otherwise specified.

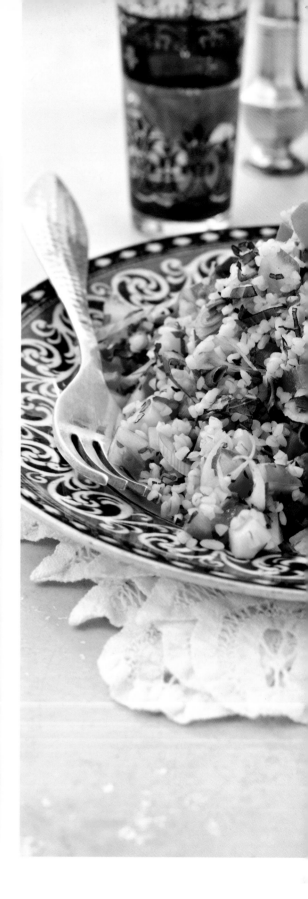

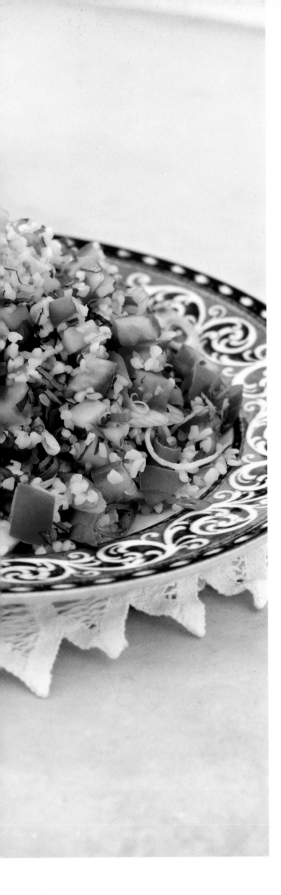

Contents

Foreword

Dear Reader,

As Slimming World's founder I've always believed passionately that our members deserve only the very best, and so I'm especially proud to introduce you to *World of Flavours*, our latest collection of fabulous Food Optimising recipes. With over 120 delicious dishes to try from around the globe, it will take you on a fascinating journey of tastes and flavours.

At Slimming World, our dedicated Consultants help thousands of new members start their weight-loss journey every week. With personal experience of struggling with excess weight, I know only too well how it feels to embark on yet another diet, losing a bit more faith in yourself each time and despairing of ever finding an answer.

Taking the first step on that journey is the hardest of all. So often, you find yourself being held back by unnecessary burdens – not just the burden of excess weight, but also the deadweight of negative beliefs, low self-esteem and guilt. Yet when you take that first step – into a Slimming World group – everything suddenly starts to get better!

The warmth of our welcome and the almost telepathic empathy and support that's at the heart of Slimming World, added to the inspiration provided by fellow slimmers succeeding beyond their wildest dreams, spark your imagination and make you realise that anything is possible. Then there's Food Optimising, a fantastic way of eating so that you're never hungry – and you're losing weight! Over 40 years on, this system is still light years ahead in its approach to nutrition and slimming psychology. Not that you think about 'nutrition' and 'psychology' when you're Food Optimising – you're too busy enjoying your food, feeling great and amazing yourself as the pounds disappear week by week.

Soon, the 'life just got better' moments start to happen again and again: the first time you see a loss on the scales, the first time your waistband feels loose, the first time someone says, 'Wow – you're looking great!', the first time you drop down a clothes size, the first time the doctor reduces your medication. Each positive experience, every encouraging or inspiring word from your Slimming World group, and each time you overcome a problem that's been holding you back, you can feel your motivation, energy and self-esteem building – each small step becomes a giant step on that road to success.

And just when you thought the service and support you get from Slimming World couldn't get any better, it does! We're constantly researching ways to make Food Optimising even easier and more effective for members, and as all our Consultants and staff know, we're always experimenting and testing new ideas then sharing the best and most effective ones so that everyone benefits.

With Extra Easy, our new Food Optimising choice, we've amazed even ourselves! It's flexible, generous and effective, just like all our Food Optimising options, with even more freedom and choices built in. And it will gently guide you to better, healthier lifestyle decisions so that once you've lost your weight, you'll keep it off for good.

At Slimming World, we always say, 'There are no strangers; only friends you have yet to meet.' If you're already a Slimming World member, you'll agree that with *World of Flavours* the best just got better. And if you have yet to join us, let your personal journey of discovery lead you to our door, where you'll always find the warmest of welcomes and the surest of successes. Together, we really can do it!

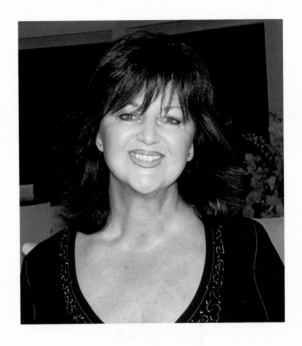

With warmest wishes

Margaret Miles-Bramwell, OBE, FRSA
Founder and Chairman

Introduction

Phileas Fogg may have travelled around the world in 80 days in his hot air balloon, but that was fiction. Here's a fact: our latest recipe collection will take you around the world in over 120 delicious dishes. We've gathered together authentic recipes from some of the world's favourite cuisines, all rich with the colours and vibrancy of the countries they represent. It's a cook's tour of global delights, and you won't even have to leave your kitchen.

Try our recipes and you'll soon be conjuring up the sunny, fresh tastes of the Mediterranean, the fragrant flavours of Thailand or the sweet and sour tang of Chinese food – whatever you fancy cooking.

The UK is famous for welcoming influences from all over the world into our national cuisine: in fact, it's said that our favourite dish is chicken tikka masala. So most of us already think of dishes like spaghetti bolognese, chilli con carne and vegetable curry as 'home cooking'. You'll find versions of classic dishes like Italian cannelloni, Greek moussaka and Indian chicken vindaloo in the book – losing weight and eating healthily needn't mean missing out on hearty family favourites.

And if your imagination takes you further afield, feel free to explore the world of flavours. Would you love to bring back memories of a sunshine holiday when it's cold and wet outside? Then try a feast of souvlakia, dolmades and tzatziki and you'll be whisked back to that beachside taverna. Recreate your favourite Indian, Chinese or Thai takeaways at a fraction of the cost, or

treat your friends to a Tex-Mex cookout – this book is full of bright ideas to fire up your tastebuds. There are plenty of ideas to appeal to your sense of culinary adventure too: if there are exotic dishes you've always wanted to make, such as a spicy Thai soup, a real Spanish paella or a Creole jambalaya, this is the book for you.

We aim to make all our recipes quick and easy to cook, so you needn't spend hours in the kitchen. And although you may be cooking dishes that originated thousands of miles away, you won't have to go to the ends of the earth to find the ingredients. If you love exploring markets and specialist food shops, that's fine – but you don't have to. Most of the dishes are based on healthy foods you find in any supermarket, like lean meat and poultry, fish, eggs, fruit, vegetables, pasta, rice and fat free dairy products. Add in a few extras like spices, herbs and seasonings – all Free Foods at Slimming World – and create a world of flavours, any time you choose.

Eat lots and still lose weight

If you're aiming to lose weight, you might now be wondering why a book of slimming recipes is encouraging you to eat your way around the world. Shouldn't you be trying to take your mind off food, instead of savouring the prospect of all these marvellous meals?

The answer is absolutely not, because this is a book of Slimming World recipes, all designed to fit in with Food Optimising, our unique way of eating well that helps you to lose weight safely and healthily and to keep it off beautifully. With over 40 years' experience of helping people overcome their weight problems, we know that the key to lasting success is to find a way of eating that allows you to celebrate your love of food and enjoy it to the full.

So instead of insisting that you stick to a straight and narrow path of banned foods and bland meals, we invite you on a journey where you decide the route. Food Optimising is flexible and generous enough to fit in with every appetite and every style of eating. French toast with strawberries for breakfast, Thai crabcakes for lunch and Moroccan lamb tagine for tea? No problem – you'll find recipes for them all in this collection, and dozens of other mouth-watering options besides.

The freedom to eat foods you like, when you like, in the quantities you like is just one of the qualities that makes Food Optimising unique. But that's not the only reason Slimming World members are encouraged to enjoy a wide range of foods and flavours to the full.

Eating a variety of foods from different food groups, especially different coloured fruit and vegetables, is a good way to ensure our diet is packed with a wide range of vitamins and minerals. And when it comes to food, variety really is 'the spice of life'; we're much more likely to make lasting changes to our eating habits if we have plenty of choice with plenty to eat.

At Slimming World, we believe that everyone deserves to enjoy delicious,

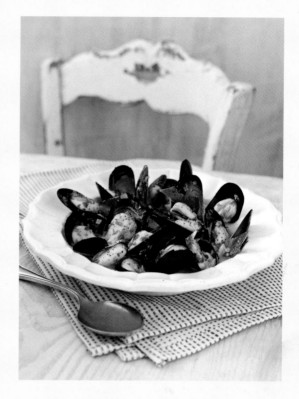

exciting, inspiring food – and that includes everyone you cook for. Because all our recipes are naturally healthy, filling and tasty, family members and friends will love them just as much as you do and they need never know you're slimming.

Above all, we know that it's possible to love your food and lose weight; our thousands of successful members show us that every week. We've created *World of Flavours* to help you discover that Food Optimising is your passport to a lifetime of healthy eating.

For details of a warm and friendly group near you, call 0844 897 8000 or visit www.slimmingworld.com

Food Optimising: the joy of food

Just leaf through the recipes in *World of Flavours*, and we're sure you'll soon be raring to go on a delicious culinary journey, exploring dishes and tastes from as far afield as China, Thailand and North America.

And if you're unhappy with your weight and would love to find a way to manage it once and for all, then you could be in for the most exciting ride of your life. That's because our recipes are all designed to fit in with Food Optimising, Slimming World's life-changing eating plan.

Most of us already know what we 'should' be doing to lose weight and eat healthily; it's just turning good intentions into real, lasting changes that's the problem.

This is where Food Optimising comes into its own. With over 40 years' experience of helping slimmers, a deep understanding of how people with weight problems feel and a passionate desire to empower them to change their lives, Slimming World is completely confident that Food Optimising has the answers, even if you've tried every kind of diet going and have been disillusioned with them all. It is said that the longest journey starts with a single step, and you could say that Food Optimising starts with a leap of faith – to put to one side everything you ever knew about 'dieting'.

If, like most of us, you have been led to believe that slimming is about eating less and going without, it can be hard to get your head around a weight-loss plan that encourages you to eat as much as you like,

whenever you like – and still lose weight every single week. That is the promise of Food Optimising.

Of course, as the saying goes, 'Nothing changes, if nothing changes'. Food Optimising requires you to make some adjustments to the way you shop, cook and eat; any weight-loss plan that claims you can slim without making any changes at all is lying to you. But these are manageable changes that are easy, and even a pleasure, to make: many Slimming World members find that they enjoy and savour their food so much more when they're Food Optimising than they did before.

So what is this amazing system all about? Well, the foundation of Food Optimising is Free Foods – a wide range of everyday, tasty, healthy foods that you can eat in unlimited amounts, whenever and wherever you like. Now, if you're in the 'dieting' mindset of set meals, banned foods and small portions, that can take a bit of swallowing!

Free Foods are fabulous
The power of Free Foods is two fold, based on sound science and a deep understanding of slimming psychology. First, Free Foods are those that have been found to have the power to satisfy our appetite and keep us feeling fuller for

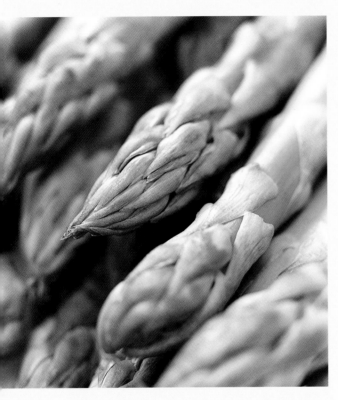

longer, without being packed with calories. Taking in fewer calories (from food) than we expend in energy (exercise and everyday activity) is the only way to lose weight, but Food Optimisers don't have to fret about counting or weighing every mouthful they eat – or even mention the 'c-word'! Filling up on Free Foods means you naturally limit your energy intake without stressing about it.

And if Free Foods are effective for weight loss, they're even more powerful in liberating slimmers from the fears and anxieties that so often sabotage success. Freed from the fear of being hungry, and from guilt about overeating – because you can't eat 'too many' Free Foods – Food Optimisers can focus on looking forward to meals, enjoying their food and generally relaxing around food, just as slim people do. (For more about Free Foods, see page 14.)

Home in on Healthy Extras

On top of that firm foundation of Free Foods, Food Optimising then becomes even more generous, flexible and realistic with the addition of Healthy Extras and Syns.

As their name suggests, Healthy Extras are foods that aren't Free, but are valuable in other ways because they are either rich in fibre or contain essential nutrients, such as calcium. Food Optimisers choose two, three or four servings of Healthy Extras each day. Wholemeal bread, soup, dried or canned fruit, cheese, breakfast cereals, milk and cereal bars are just some of the foods on the Healthy Extras list that can be eaten either with meals or as snacks. (For more about Healthy Extras, see pages 15–16.)

Syns spell success

And then, on top of all those Free Foods and Healthy Extras, there are Syns. They come last, but by no means least, because although Syns account for only a small percentage of your daily food intake when you're Food Optimising, they can make all the difference to your long-term success. Foods that are high in Syns are typically those we need to limit if we want to lose weight and for good health: things like fatty, sugary and processed foods, and alcohol. Syns aren't essential for nutrition, but if you just love chocolate or have a serious biscuit habit, they're pretty important to you! So, every day, Food

Optimisers have between 5 and 15 Syns to use whenever and however they like. In fact, you could say Syns are the icing on the cake – quite literally, if that's how you choose to spend them. (For more on Syns, see page 16.)

Freedom to eat and freedom to choose, with just a few checks and balances to keep weight loss progressing healthily and easily – this freedom is at the heart of Food Optimising's success.

So how do you mix and match your Free Foods, Healthy Extras and Syns into meals every day? Here again, it's all about freedom and choice; if you're expecting to be handed a diet sheet, we're sorry to disappoint you!

Depending on which foods you love to eat and how you prefer to plan your meals, there are five choices, or styles of menu, you can follow when you're Food Optimising:

- Original,
- Green,
- Extra Easy,
- Success Express,
- Free2Go.

Each choice is described opposite and, of course, when you join Slimming World you have the chance to explore each one to find out which works best for you. You needn't stick to one choice for ever, or even for a whole week: it's all about being flexible so that you stay positive, focused and motivated to make each week a fabulous weight-loss week.

With so many foods to choose from, and so much flexibility around meals, you can see just how easy it is to fit Food

FOOD OPTIMISING CHOICES AT A GLANCE

Original choice

Roast dinners, a tasty burger, full English breakfast or a mixed grill: if you love hearty meals like these, then Food Optimising's Original choice is for you. They don't sound like 'slimming' meals? Prepared the Slimming World way, they certainly are. Satisfying protein-rich foods, such as lean meat, poultry, fish and seafood, are all Free Foods on Original, along with all fresh fruit and nearly all vegetables, plus eggs and some dairy products such as fat free yogurt or fromage frais. Add delicious daily Healthy Extras, such as wholemeal bread, potatoes, high-fibre breakfast cereals and cheese or milk, then decide how to use your Syns for the day.

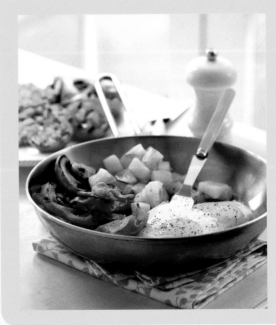

Green choice

Are your favourite meals a heap of pasta with sauce, tasty vegetable chilli with rice or a huge jacket potato with beans and cheese? Then Food Optimising's Green choice is for you. Yes, you really can eat comforting, carbohydrate-rich foods including pasta, potatoes, rice, couscous, beans and pulses and lose weight beautifully, as well as many other Free Foods, such as all fresh fruit and vegetables, eggs and dairy products like fat free yogurt or fromage frais. Love fish and meat too? Just add them as Healthy Extras, or choose wholemeal bread, high-fibre breakfast cereals and cheese or milk to provide even more energy, fibre, vitamins and minerals, then choose your Syns.

Extra Easy

As all the Food Optimising choices are the easiest you'll find anywhere, a choice called Extra Easy has a lot to live up to – and it does! At every Extra Easy meal you take your pick from a long list of Free Foods from both the Green and Original choices, filling your plate on a two-thirds Free, one-third Superfree basis (go back for seconds or thirds if you like). Have two Healthy Extras a day, plus your Syns, and just watch your motivation soar as those pounds roll away.

Success Express

We all have times when we need a boost, and Success Express is just the ticket if you want to move your weight loss up a gear. With Success Express, you have three satisfying meals a day based on Superfree and Free Foods, on a two-thirds Superfree, one-third Free principle. You can choose Free Foods from the Original or Green list – both at the same meal if you like. And there's still no need to weigh and measure! You have your Healthy Extras and Syns, as with the other choices, and snack on Superfree Foods, so you can be confident your weight loss is speeding along, without worrying about going hungry.

Free2Go

If managing their weight is an issue, the last thing teenagers need is a plan that gets them hung up on calorie-counting or that isolates them from their friends. So Slimming World's Free2Go was developed specially for young people aged 11–15: it allows unlimited Original and Green Free Foods, a long list of Healthy Extras, most in unlimited quantities, and a small number of high-fat or high-sugar choices each day, with the focus on making 'cool swaps' towards healthier foods.

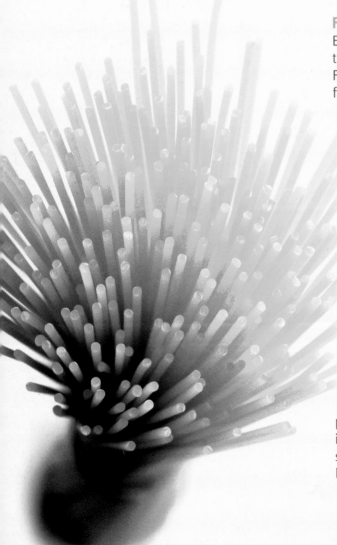

Optimising into your lifestyle, rather than the other way round. Eating with the family, eating out, going to work, going on holiday, having 'hungry days' and busy days – whatever you're doing, you can be confident that you can still Food Optimise successfully. And if you do have a tricky situation to deal with, the support and ideas you'll get from your Slimming World Consultant and fellow members each week will soon help you to find a way through. You will also find stacks of support on the website, LifelineOnline, which is free of charge for members.

Freedom to explore, choices to enjoy, flexibility to suit your needs, and just enough controls to ensure you stay safe and have a great time – if Food Optimising were a round-the-world trip, it would be the best ever. And if you want to lose your excess baggage and travel light for the rest of your life, it's definitely the best ticket you can buy.

Free Foods

Eat more and still lose weight? It sounds too good to be true – but when you're Food Optimising, it becomes a fabulous fact of life.

The secret of being able to eat until you're full at every meal, yet slim down steadily every week, is Free Foods: foods you can eat in unlimited amounts, whenever you like. No measuring, weighing or counting – no worries! Free Foods are at the heart of Food Optimising and they are the masterstroke that makes the Slimming World way of eating so generous, flexible and effective. Yet although they work like magic, there is nothing magic about them; they are everyday foods that you'll enjoy cooking and eating every day. The reason why Food Optimisers can pile up their plates and still lose weight is that Free Foods are particularly good at satisfying appetite, and are also relatively low in calories, weight for weight. So filling up on Free Foods is a win-win situation: it means never having to fear feeling hungry, and never having to worry that by satisfying your appetite you are sabotaging your weight loss. Two of the biggest obstacles slimmers face – destroyed at one stroke!

On the Free Foods list you'll find protein-rich foods like lean meat, poultry, fish and eggs, and starchy foods like pasta and potatoes, rice, beans and grains. That's because scientific studies have found that both protein-rich foods and starchy foods are more satiating (good at satisfying appetite) than foods that are high in fat and sugar.

You'll also find lots of foods like fruit and vegetables, which are low in energy density – in other words they have fewer calories, weight for weight, than other foods. These are a slimmer's best friend because they are filling without stacking up the calories.

Speed Foods: Some Free Foods are even lower in energy density than others in their group, and at Slimming World these are known as Speed Foods. Focusing on Speed Foods can give your weight loss a kick-start, although no individual food can be said to be 'fattening' or 'slimming' – it's your overall diet that counts.

Superfree Foods: Some foods are not just Free, but Superfree! This means that they are Free on both the Green and the Original choice, so they are great to fill up with,

snack on throughout the day or to add to meals. They include all fresh and frozen fruit, most vegetables, eggs, some fat free dairy products and vegetable proteins like Quorn and tofu. Superfree Foods are at the heart of the Success Express choice, which is designed to give your weight loss a special boost (see page 13), and of our new Extra Easy plan (see page 13). As thousands of Slimming World members have already found, Extra Easy is our most liberating choice ever, allowing you to choose Free Foods from the Green and Original choices at every meal.

If the recipes in *World of Flavours* whet your appetite (and of course they will!) you'll be amazed how many foods from all around the globe are Free for Food Optimisers. On the Green choice, fill up on rice with Indian meals, pasta with an Italian feast, or couscous with a luxurious Moroccan tagine. On Original, take your pick from the meat, fish and shellfish counter and add your choice of spices, herbs and seasonings – they're all Free on every choice. And don't forget your fruit and vegetables: healthy eating guidelines recommend that we eat at least five servings a day, but Food Optimisers regularly find they eat more – there are no limits, except your imagination.

Healthy Extras

Food Optimising is all about balancing freedom with a light touch of control.

> **Free Foods are at the heart of Food Optimising and they are the masterstroke that makes the Slimming World way of eating so generous, flexible and effective**

Healthy Extras are the checks in the system, there to ensure that Food Optimisers enjoy foods from the key food groups, and important elements of a balanced diet every day.

Unlike Free Foods, Healthy Extras are eaten in measured portions, and they too can be eaten any time of day – with meals or as snacks – however you like to eat. The generous list of Healthy Extras you can choose from every day is made up of foods that are high in fibre, or in other nutrients, vitamins and minerals needed for optimum health, especially calcium.

Fibre-rich foods are among the most powerful appetite-satisfiers, as well as keeping your digestive system healthy and helping to protect against many diseases.

Calcium is needed to build strong bones and teeth, and to help nerves, muscle and blood to function properly. Research has also found that calcium may play a role in metabolising fat and so is potentially extra-helpful for weight loss. If you don't like or can't eat dairy products, there are soya-based alternatives to choose from.

Some Healthy Extras appear on the Green, Original and Extra Easy lists. They include dairy products such as milk and cheese and high-fibre foods, such as wholemeal bread, breakfast cereals and cereal bars.

On the Green choice, Healthy Extras also include lean meat, poultry and fish, and on the Original choice, they include wholemeal pasta, potatoes, pulses and beans.

The number of Healthy Extras you have each day depends which Food Optimising choice you are following: choose three or four a day on the Green, Original and Success Express choices, and two a day on the Extra Easy choice.

Healthy Extras make Food Optimising more convenient for everyday meals and more flexible for eating out; for instance, on the Original choice you can use wholemeal bread as a Healthy Extra to make a tuna sandwich for work, or in a restaurant you can order new potatoes as a Healthy Extra with your gammon steak. On the Green choice, you could have grilled chicken with a big pasta salad, or prawns on your jacket potato.

Syns

'Syn' may sound like something that you have to confess to, or repent of – but at Slimming World there's nothing sinful about Syns!

Synergy is the super powerful effect that individual elements have when they combine to achieve more than they could on their own. We think of it as $2 + 2 = 5$!

Syns take the guilt out of enjoying a chocolate fix, a drink after work or a packet of crisps.

Slimming World is just full of synergies happening all over the place: Food Optimising, Image Therapy (see pages 18–21) and Body Magic (see pages 22–25), for example, are all effective on their own, but combine them and they're sensational! And part of that synergy is Syns.

In Food Optimising terms, Syns are the third element, with Free Foods and Healthy Extras, which creates a completely healthy and effective eating plan that you can live

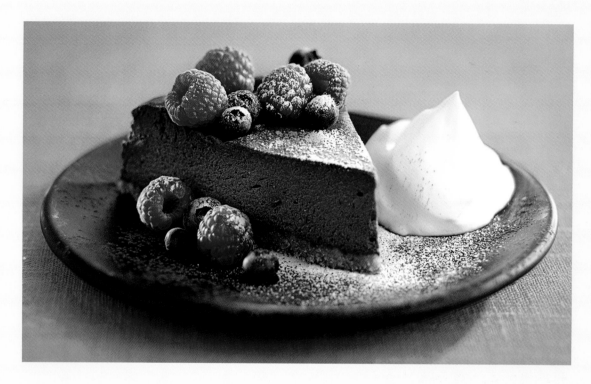

with in the long term. They take the guilt out of enjoying a chocolate fix, a drink after work or a packet of crisps. You can enjoy your Syns as snacks, or to make meals even more enticing; there's no need to miss out on little extras like ketchup on your burger or cream on your strawberries.

Each day, Food Optimisers decide how many Syns they would like to use, on top of all their Free Foods and Healthy Extra choices.

All foods that aren't Free or Healthy Extras have a Syn value. You probably won't be surprised to find that a lot of foods that are high in Syns are the fatty, sugary, processed foods that we are all advised to eat less of, whether we wish to lose weight or not. Fast foods, many ready-meals, snacks, pies, cakes and desserts, along with alcohol, are some of the foods

that are high in Syns because they pack a lot of calories for their weight, meaning that they are 'energy dense' and easy to overeat.

Free Foods, by contrast, are generally basic, unprocessed foods like fruit and vegetables, meat and fish, eggs, pasta and rice, so filling up on Free Foods and counting your Syns is a great way to ensure that you naturally eat more fresh, basic foods and less fatty and sugary foods.

But don't for a moment think that means feeling deprived. As you'll see from the recipes in this book, you can enjoy creamy curries, hearty casseroles, burgers and tasty desserts, and still stay well within your Syns allowance each day. It's a question of cooking and eating the Slimming World way – making small changes that add up to a life-changing difference.

Image Therapy: group support

As soon as you walk through the doors of any Slimming World group, you can feel there's something special going on: there's a warmth, friendliness and liveliness that shines out, which you just don't find anywhere else.

It doesn't happen by accident; group support is at the heart of Slimming World, and for over 40 years the company has been passionately devoted to providing the best possible service for members every week.

The process that harnesses the power of the group every week and turns it into dazzling successes is called IMAGE Therapy. It stands for Individual Motivation And Group Experience, but some think of it as Inspiration Makes A Great Evening! It's an opportunity for members, guided by their Consultant, to share their highs and lows, celebrate each other's achievements and offer support when things aren't going so well. Everyone has a chance to contribute, and members find that hearing about someone else's week gives them all the ideas they need to change their own.

The support continues between group meetings too; members buddy up to become 'Lifelines' for each other by texting, emailing or phoning during the week, and those who are online have exclusive free access to a website with services such as interactive food diaries, a personalised progress chart and searchable recipe archive, with loads of information and inspiration on top.

Despite what you might have heard about other slimming clubs, there is never any humiliation, ridicule, judgement or embarrassing revelations in Slimming World groups. No one's weight is revealed to the group; weighing happens in private, but celebration of weight lost is very public indeed. Even when a member has a weight gain (and it happens to almost everyone at some point on their journey), the support remains positive and motivating. Far from being made to feel guilty or – heaven forbid – being punished for gaining weight, at Slimming World members are praised for coming to the group when it would have been tempting to stay away, and encouraged to have a better week, starting today.

And the same applies for members who are returning to their group after a time away; no matter where they are with their weight, each one is welcomed just as warmly as the first time round.

Every Slimming World member sets their own weight-loss target each week and there's no pressure to decide a final target when you first join. One milestone that everyone is encouraged to aim for, though, is called Club 10, which you achieve when you've lost 10 per cent of your starting weight and maintained that weight, or lost more, for 10 weeks. You're rewarded with a free week's membership (and wild applause from the group!), but even more

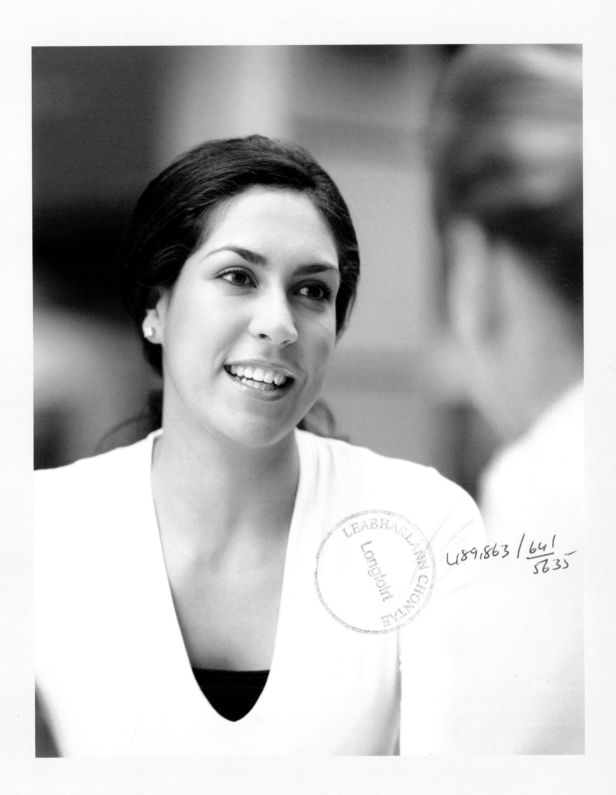

importantly if you're overweight, a 10 per cent weight loss is enough to start reaping real benefits to health, in terms of lowered blood pressure, reduced risk of developing conditions like heart disease and type 2 diabetes, and less strain on joints.

One of the criticisms we hear about slimming clubs is that once you've lost the weight, they lose interest in you. The absolute opposite is true at Slimming World. Members who have reached their personal target weight are vital to the life of each group, so much so that once you've reached your target you can attend Slimming World free of charge every week for ever, as long as you stay in your target range. Target members have a huge amount to contribute to the group, both as an inspiration to other members and as a source of experience. And because we know that staying slim can be just as hard as losing weight, target members are encouraged to continue coming to keep their own motivation high too.

Children and young adults

Over the years, Slimming World has prided itself on being a pioneer in many areas, and is always looking for opportunities to help even more people to solve their weight problems for good – even if it means tackling situations that others shy away from.

For example, it's been clear for some time that children in the UK are becoming heavier, less active and more prone to weight-related conditions such as type 2 diabetes. It's been described as the biggest public health issue of our time. Many experts agree that the problem needs to be addressed urgently, but because young people's weight is such a sensitive issue, very little practical help has so far been available.

So Slimming World's family-friendly programme represents a real breakthrough in helping young people (from 11 to 15) manage their weight if they need to. In a membership package designed just for them, young people can attend Slimming World free of charge, as long as they're accompanied by a parent or guardian who is a member (this is essential, because encouraging the whole family to change lifestyle habits is so often the key to success).

For Slimming World's young members – and thousands have joined since the scheme was introduced – the emphasis isn't on weight loss, but on plenty of praise and support for taking on board positive lifestyle changes. A specially created version of Food Optimising, called Free2Go (see page 13), is a super-simple way of eating with no counting and measuring – just plenty of everyday, tasty foods and suggestions for making swaps from less healthy to healthier options. Feedback from young members and their families has been fantastic and many have managed to control their weight effectively without ever feeling that they are 'on a

> **Food Optimising is an ideal way for breastfeeding women to enjoy a varied, healthy diet at this crucial time, while regaining their figure safely.**

diet' or missing out on teenage life. Along with boosted self-confidence and new-found energy, they're also laying down a foundation of healthy habits that will stand them in good stead for life.

Support for mums

Many new mums join Slimming World to lose surplus pounds that have crept on during pregnancy. Food Optimising is an ideal way for breast-feeding women to enjoy a varied, healthy diet that supplies all the extra energy and nutrients needed at this crucial time, while regaining their figure safely and steadily. And our care for the family starts even earlier, as Slimming World is the only national slimming club to support pregnant women as they balance the needs of their growing baby with managing their own weight gain. This is so important, because putting on too much weight increases the likelihood of complications during pregnancy, such as gestational diabetes or high blood pressure, and interventions during the birth.

Working with the Royal College of Midwives, Slimming World has developed a supportive, positive policy to help women at this special time in their lives. Members who wish to continue attending Slimming World during their pregnancy are required to get the consent of their midwife, who will make any recommendations on managing their weight safely.

Slimming World and the NHS

Improving the nation's health is also at the heart of another pioneering Slimming World service, Slimming World on Referral.

We are proud to be working with over 50 Primary Care Trusts to provide Slimming World membership free of charge to patients who would benefit from losing weight and are referred to their local group by their GP or practice nurse. Research that Slimming World has conducted and published in scientific journals shows that our members lose weight safely and steadily – and at a fraction of the cost that health authorities might spend on drugs or surgery.

With the Slimming World on Referral scheme, members receive 12 weeks' free membership at their local group, after which their GP may refer them for a further 12 weeks or more, or they may choose to continue their membership, paying for themselves. Many do continue as paying members, so delighted are they with the results they've been able to achieve in a relatively short time. The rate at which you lose weight with Slimming World varies; some members enjoy big weight losses in the first weeks, which is quite natural. Generally, it averages out to a steady 450–900 grams (1–2 pounds) a week in the long run, which is ideal for sustainable, healthy weight loss.

Slimming World's success with its family-friendly plan and Slimming World on Referral shows that the unique formula works for young and not so young, whatever their motivation for slimming.

But whatever leads them through Slimming World's doors, every member will find the same magical mix of ingredients: a warm welcome, a friendly, dedicated Consultant and the unique synergy of Food Optimising, Body Magic and Image Therapy – the heart of Slimming World.

Body Magic: active for life

Losing weight and keeping it off is all about the 'energy equation': taking in less energy from food than we spend in activity. Food Optimising takes care of the 'energy in' side of the equation; as we've already seen, it's a fabulously effective way of limiting your calorie intake naturally.

All the research shows, though, that working on the 'energy out' side of the equation, by becoming more active, can really help your weight loss and especially maintenance of your weight loss. Adding three to four moderate exercise sessions a week to a healthy eating plan will help you lose around 450–900 grams (1–2 pounds) a month more than you would by dieting alone – that's an extra 5½–11 kilograms (12–24 pounds) a year.

And that's quite apart from the benefits that moderate, regular exercise has for your general health. Study after study shows that people who are more active have a lower risk of heart disease and certain cancers, including breast cancer; they are likely to have lower blood pressure, stronger muscles, bones and joints, and are less likely to develop type 2 diabetes.

In addition to the physical benefits, exercising regularly can also have a powerful positive effect on your energy levels, quality of sleep, self-confidence and mood – which is extremely valuable when you're trying to make long-lasting lifestyle changes.

So all in all, combining some moderate activity with your Food Optimising is a sure-fire way to boost your weight loss. As you'd expect from Slimming World, we thought long and hard about how best to help members become more active, in the way that works best for them and employs all of Slimming World's famous strengths – freedom, choices, flexibility and support.

And what we came up with was magic! Body Magic, in fact. It's our way of describing the synergy that's created by combining Food Optimising with the right kind of moderate activity – the kind that's right for you.

There's no big secret to Body Magic; it's as simple as encouraging people to increase the amount of activity they do each day on a regular basis.

There's no big secret to Body Magic; it's as simple as encouraging people to increase the amount of activity they do each day on a regular basis, and to recognise and reward their efforts when they do. It's not about gym membership, intensive workouts or team sports – although if you enjoy any of those things, that's fine and you'll be applauded.

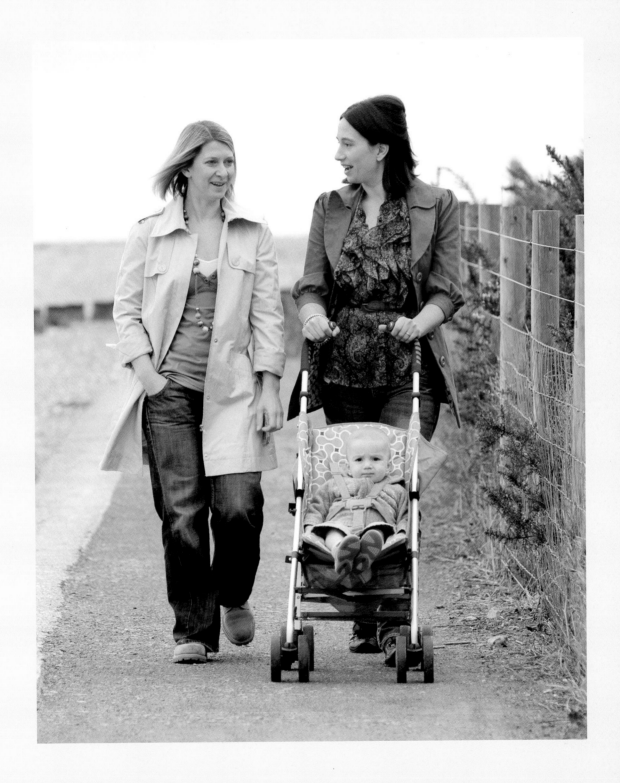

For people who aren't sporty, though (and that's most of us), Body Magic is about finding types of activity you enjoy, and can stick to, and are able to build into their way of life. You can't store up the benefits of exercise, so in the long term it's not very helpful to start an exercise regime with a spurt of enthusiasm, only for it to fizzle out in a week or two. Research shows that people who see exercising as an intrinsic part of their everyday routine – as natural as cleaning their teeth – reap the most benefits over time.

The fact is, though, that if you have never exercised, or feel just too old, unfit or heavy to do so, getting motivated feels like a mountain to climb. Slimming World understands this only too well, so Body Magic starts where you are now – on the path from a sedentary to an active lifestyle – not where you should be.

Just as Food Optimising starts with challenging conventional wisdom about dieting, Body Magic starts with some myth-busting about exercise. First is that you don't need to do a tremendous amount of activity for it to be effective: a chunk of 15 minutes at a time is fine. Second, the speed you move at doesn't make much difference; of course, if you run a certain distance, you'll get there quicker than if you walk briskly, but the energy you expend will be about the same. It's moving your body around that counts, and the heavier the body, the greater the energy you expend – so if you have a lot of weight to lose, you have potentially even more to gain by getting active.

Brisk walking is probably the activity that's most popular with Slimming World members, and it's easy to see why: it's free, it's easy, and you can do it anywhere, any time, on your own or in company. It's also one of the best all-round forms of exercise for fat burning, improving your heart's fitness and strengthening your bones.

But the main thing about any exercise plan is to enjoy it; having fun is more than half the battle in becoming a regular exerciser. So all around the country you'll find Slimming World members swimming, dancing, doing aerobics, cycling, jogging and playing sports from badminton to water polo – and many of them have amazed themselves at what they've been able to achieve.

Another myth about exercise is that what we do every day – housework, gardening, cleaning the car – doesn't count as 'proper' exercise. If you put your back into it, it does! Even if you can't get outside, an hour's spring-cleaning is just as good as a 30-minute brisk walk.

And exercising that has a purpose can be even easier to fit into a busy day: cycling to work, walking to the sandwich shop instead of going to the canteen, or getting off the bus a stop earlier, can all help you become more active, more often.

So how does all this fit into Slimming World's Body Magic programme?

As with Food Optimising, it's all about members setting their own goals, choosing how they want to reach them, and being supported every step of the way. Each week, members are encouraged to set Body Magic goals that they note down in a private FIT Log (FIT stands for Frequency, Intensity and Time). This might be, for instance, 'walk 30 minutes a day' or 'dance

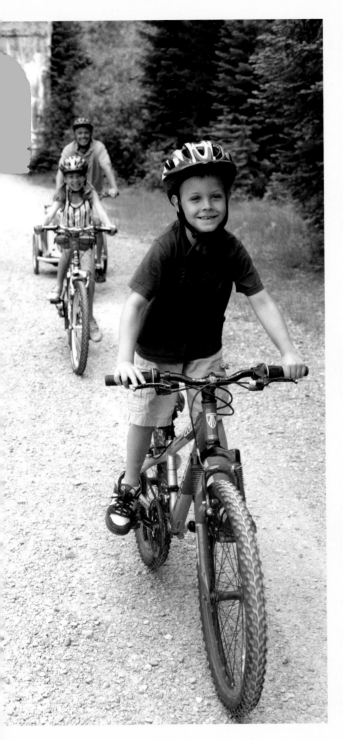

to activity video for a total of an hour this week'.

As they gradually build up the amount of time they spend on activity, members can work towards Body Magic awards, which are earned at different stages:

- Bronze, when you're active for at least 45 minutes each week, spread over at least three days and maintained for four weeks or more.
- Silver, which you reach four weeks after building up to six 15-minute sessions of activity each week, spread over three to five days and maintained for four weeks.
- Gold, achieved when you are being active for ten 15-minute sessions a week, spread over five days or more and maintained for eight weeks. This is the level the Government recommends for maintaining good health.
- Platinum, when exercise and activity are automatic and regular in your weekly routine and you can't imagine life without them.

There's no timetable for achieving each stage; just like Food Optimising, members make progress at their own pace. Some find that just the inspiration and encouragement they find in their group is enough to turn them from couch potatoes to enthusiastic exercisers quite quickly; others take a more 'scenic route' on their journey. Everyone enjoys the same congratulations and applause when they reach another milestone. And everyone is moving towards the same destination: a fitter, healthier body for life.

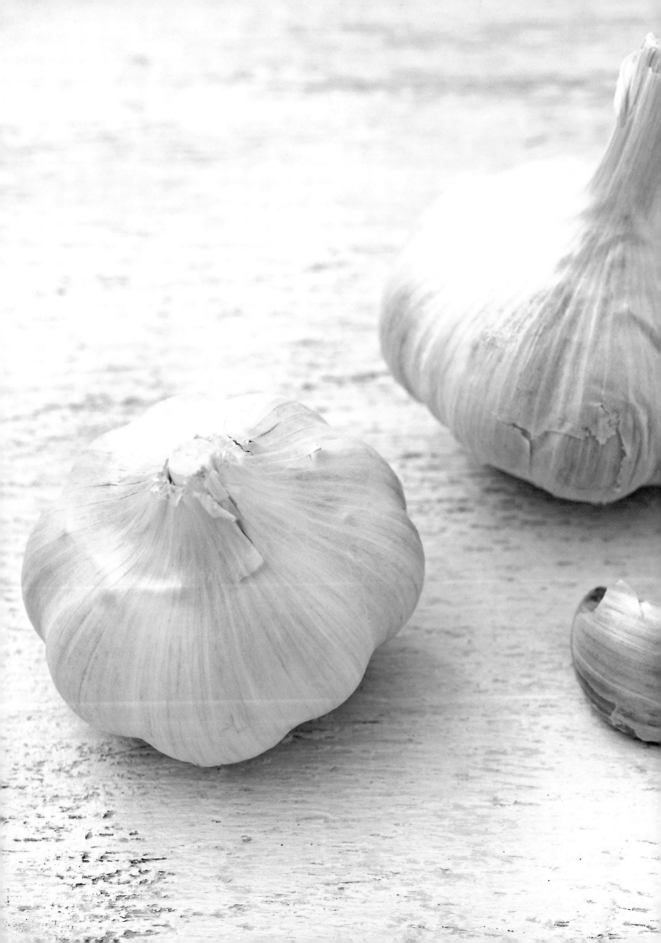

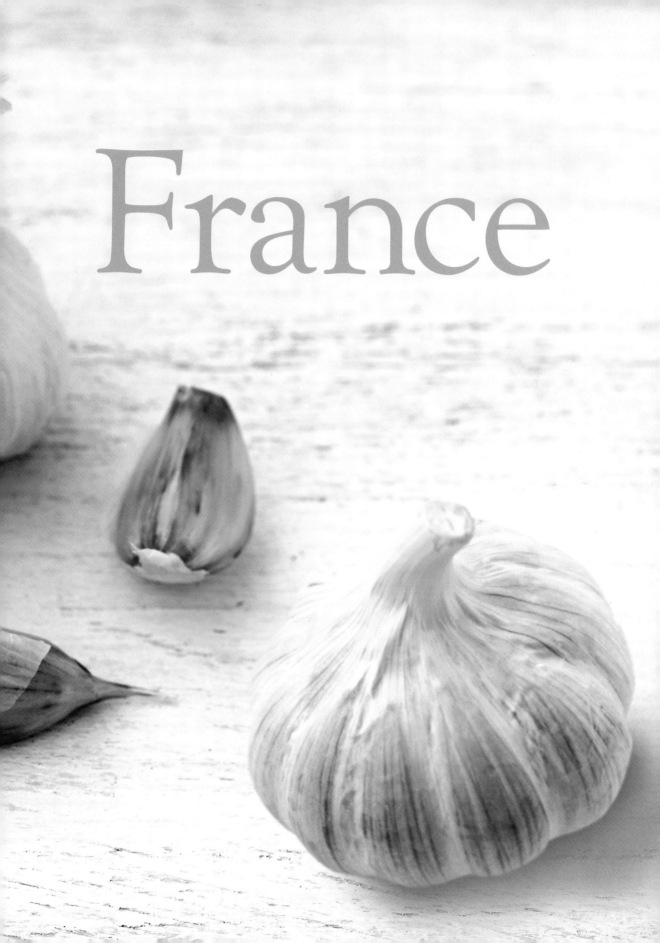

France

Potage au cresson

SERVES 4

EASY Ⓥ ❄

Syns per serving
Extra Easy: Free
Green: Free
Original: 1

Preparation time 20 minutes
Cooking time 35–40 minutes

low calorie cooking spray
2 garlic cloves, peeled and crushed
1 leek, trimmed and roughly chopped
1 thyme sprig
1 medium potato, peeled and diced
1.5 litres/2½ pints vegetable stock
250g/9oz watercress, finely chopped
salt and freshly ground black pepper
a pinch of finely grated nutmeg
150g/5oz fat free natural fromage frais

TO SERVE
a few watercress sprigs

The sharp flavour of watercress adds some zing to this soup. For a chunkier version you can omit the blending process and just stir in the fromage frais before serving.

Spray a heavy-based saucepan with low calorie cooking spray and place over a medium heat. Add the garlic and leek and sauté for 6–8 minutes until softened.

Add the thyme, potato and stock and bring to the boil. Simmer for 15–20 minutes and then add the chopped watercress. Simmer for 3–4 minutes, season well and add the nutmeg. Transfer to a food processor and blend until smooth, adding the fromage frais gradually, until well blended.

To serve, ladle into warmed soup plates and top each serving with a watercress sprig.

Spinach and potato gratin

SERVES 4

EASY Ⓥ ❋

Syns per serving
Extra Easy: 3½
Green: 3½
Original: 9½

Preparation time 10 minutes
Cooking time 30 minutes

600g/1lb 6oz potatoes, peeled and
thinly sliced
500g/1lb 2oz spinach, trimmed
low calorie cooking spray
100g/3½oz reduced fat Cheddar cheese,
grated
salt and freshly ground black pepper
4 tomatoes, sliced
3 eggs, beaten
200g/7oz fat free natural yogurt

TO SERVE
a crisp green salad

For a spicy version of this dish, stir a tablespoon of medium curry powder, a finely diced red chilli and 4 tablespoons of finely chopped coriander into the egg and yogurt mixture before whisking it and pouring it over the vegetables.

Preheat the oven to 180°C/Gas 4. Cook the potatoes in lightly salted boiling water for about 5 minutes and then drain well. Meanwhile, cook the spinach in boiling water for 1–2 minutes, drain and squeeze out any excess water.

Spray a large casserole dish with low calorie cooking spray and line the bottom with half the potatoes, then cover with the spinach and half the Cheddar, seasoning each layer well.

Cover with the rest of the potatoes and arrange the tomato slices on top. Sprinkle with the remaining cheese. In a separate bowl, whisk together the eggs and yogurt and season well. Pour over the dish. Bake for about 30 minutes. Remove from the oven and serve with a crisp green salad.

Normandy onion soup

SERVES 4

EASY Ⓥ ❄

Syns per serving
Extra Easy: ½
Original: ½
Green: ½

Preparation time 15 minutes
Cooking time 35–40 minutes

low calorie cooking spray
6 medium onions, peeled and thinly
sliced
1 garlic clove, peeled and thinly sliced
1 tbsp chopped thyme leaves
100ml/3½fl oz Normandy cider
900ml/1½ pints vegetable stock or
water
salt and freshly ground black pepper
chopped flat-leaf parsley

Using cider from Normandy makes for the special flavour in this hearty onion soup. You can use dry or sweet cider if you can't get your hands on the French stuff.

Spray a heavy-based saucepan with low calorie cooking spray. Sauté the onions and garlic for 20–25 minutes over a low heat, until golden brown.

Stir well then add the thyme, cider and stock or water. Bring to the boil and simmer for 10–15 minutes. Add seasoning to the soup, scatter with chopped parsley and serve immediately.

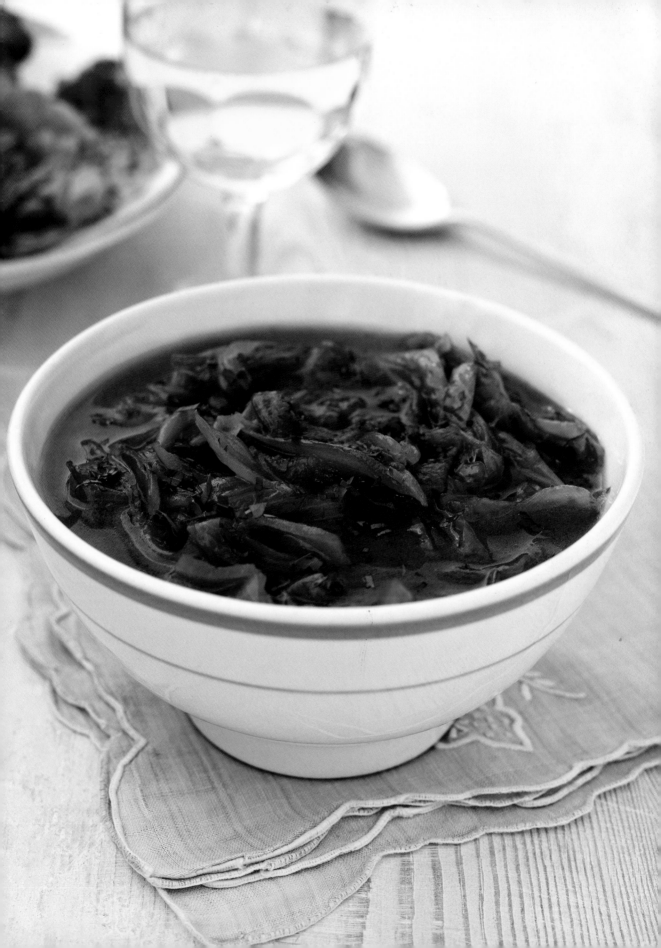

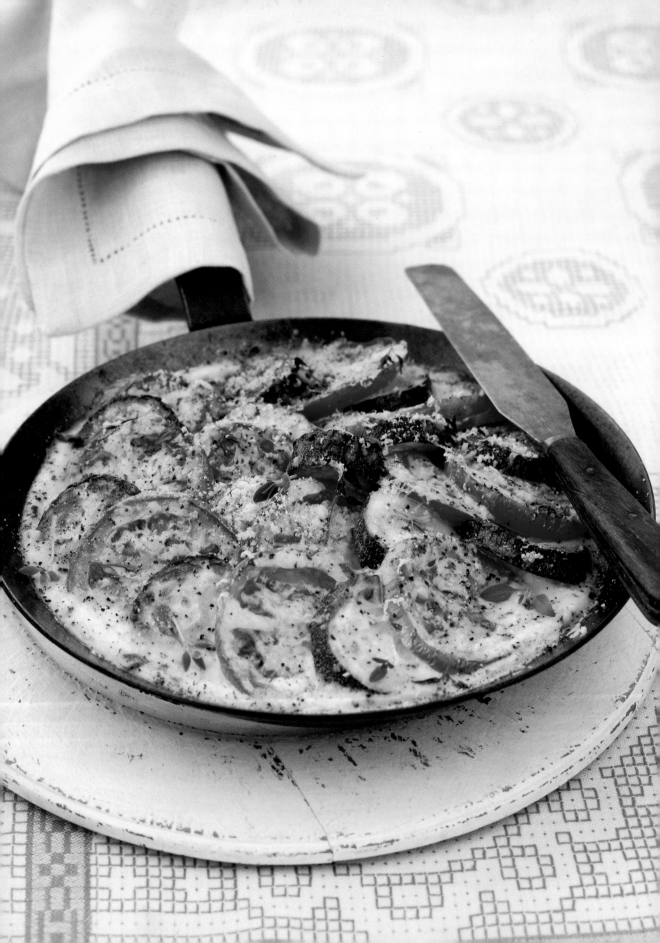

Tomato and courgette flan

SERVES 4

EASY Ⓥ ✳

Syns per serving
Extra Easy: 1
Original: 1
Green: 1

Preparation time 20 minutes
Cooking time about 45 minutes

low calorie cooking spray
2 courgettes, cut into 5mm/¼in slices
3 eggs
1 tbsp chopped thyme leaves
1 garlic clove, peeled and crushed
100g/3½oz quark
25g/1oz reduced fat Cheddar cheese,
grated
salt and freshly ground black pepper
4 medium tomatoes, cut into
5mm/¼in slices

TO SERVE
a crisp salad or steamed green
vegetables

This savoury flan is very versatile as you can vary the basic vegetables in the dish to suit your taste or to ring a change.

Preheat the oven to 200°C/Gas 6. Spray a large non-stick frying pan with low calorie cooking spray and place over a high heat. Add the courgettes and cook for 2–3 minutes on each side, until lightly browned. Remove from the heat.

Beat the eggs in a large bowl, stir in the thyme, garlic, quark and half the Cheddar and season well.

Lightly spray a medium, shallow ovenproof frying pan or flan dish with low calorie cooking spray and pour in half the egg mixture.

Arrange the courgettes and tomatoes over the egg mixture in alternating slices, pour over the remaining egg mixture and top with the remaining cheese. Cook in the oven for 30–35 minutes until golden and set. Serve warm or at room temperature with a crisp green salad or steamed green vegetables.

Celeriac dauphinois

Usually made with potatoes and cream, this celeriac version of a classic French dish has all the flavour of the original, but without the fat.

SERVES 4

EASY Ⓥ ❄

Syns per serving
Extra Easy: Free
Original: Free
Green: Free

Preparation time 15 minutes
Cooking time about 1 hour

low calorie cooking spray
800g/1lb 12oz celeriac, peeled
and cut into thin sticks
2 large onions, peeled,
halved and thinly sliced
150g/5oz quark
200ml/7fl oz vegetable stock
3 tsp garlic salt
freshly ground black pepper

TO SERVE
chopped flat-leaf parsley

Preheat the oven to 200°C/Gas 6. Spray a medium-sized ovenproof dish with low calorie cooking spray. Arrange half the celeriac in the dish and cover with the onions. Top with the remaining celeriac.

In a large bowl, beat the quark until smooth and stir in the stock and garlic salt to make a smooth mixture. Season well with pepper and pour over the top of the celeriac and onions. Spray lightly with low calorie cooking spray and bake in the oven for 50–60 minutes. (If the top is browning too quickly, cover with foil.)

Remove from the oven and allow the dish to rest for a few minutes then garnish with chopped parsley before serving.

Ratatouille

SERVES 4

EASY (V) (❄)

Syns per serving
Extra Easy: Free
Original: Free
Green: Free

Preparation time 10 minutes
Cooking time 25 minutes

low calorie cooking spray
2 onions, peeled and chopped
1 aubergine, halved and sliced
2 large courgettes, halved and sliced
1 red pepper, deseeded and cubed
1 yellow pepper, deseeded and cubed
2 garlic cloves, peeled and crushed
400g can chopped tomatoes
salt and freshly ground black pepper
4 tbsp chopped flat-leaf parsley

Traditional ratatouille is a mix of garlic, onions, peppers, courgettes and aubergine braised with lots and lots of olive oil. It's healthy, but not exactly low fat. This Syn-free version has all the flavour, without the oil!

Spray a large non-stick frying pan with low calorie cooking spray and place over a medium heat. Add the onions, aubergine, courgettes, peppers and garlic and stir-fry for a few minutes.

Add the tomatoes, season and stir well. Cover tightly and simmer for 15–20 minutes until all the vegetables are cooked and tender.

Remove from the heat and stir in the chopped parsley before serving.

Moules marinières

Fresh, live mussels are widely available in fishmongers and at the fish counters of many supermarkets. They are quick to cook and are perfect for last-minute entertaining.

SERVES 4

EASY

Syns per serving
Extra Easy: 1
Original: 1
Green: 8

Preparation time 10 minutes
Cooking time 5–6 minutes

2kg/4lb 8oz mussels
6 garlic cloves, peeled and finely chopped
4 shallots, peeled and very finely chopped
1 bay leaf
1 tbsp crushed fennel seeds
100ml/3½fl oz dry white wine
200ml/7fl oz fish stock
4 tbsp fat free natural fromage frais
salt and freshly ground black pepper
4 tbsp finely chopped flat-leaf parsley

Scrub and remove any 'beards' from the mussels and discard any mussels that are open.

Place the mussels, garlic, shallots, bay leaf, fennel seeds, white wine and stock in a large saucepan and place over a high heat. Cover tightly and cook for 5–6 minutes, shaking the pan frequently, until the mussels have opened. Discard any that remain closed.

Drain the mussels, reserving any juices, and divide between four warmed bowls. Mix the fromage frais into the reserved juices and spoon over the mussels. Season, garnish with the parsley and serve immediately.

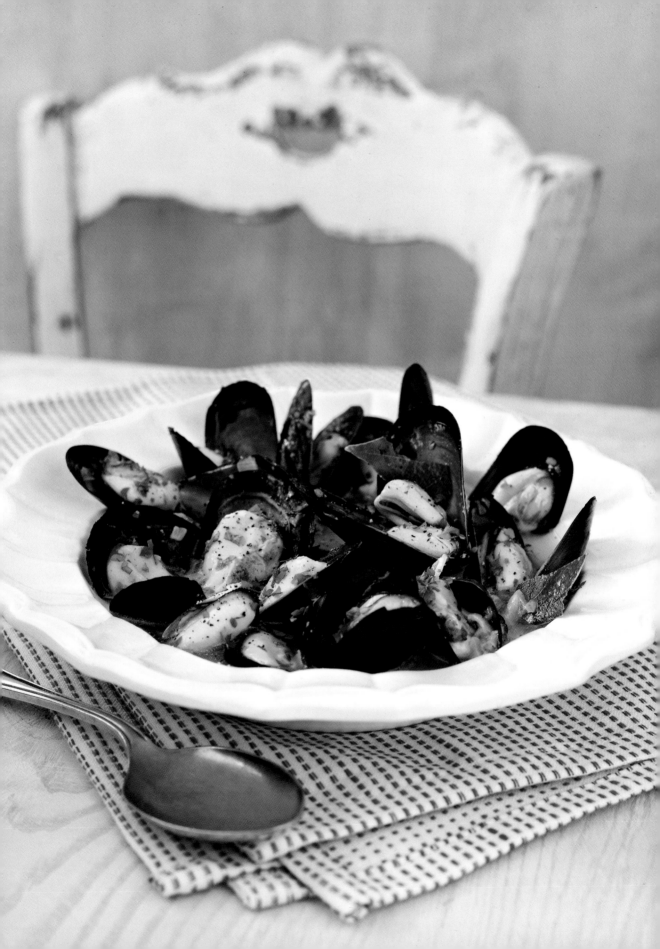

Tuna niçoise salad

SERVES 4

REALLY EASY

Syns per serving
Extra Easy: ½
Original: ½
Green: 6

Preparation time 15 minutes

200g/7oz green beans, trimmed
2 little gem lettuces, leaves separated
100g/3½oz each of red and yellow
cherry tomatoes, halved
1 red onion, peeled and thinly sliced
400g/14oz canned tuna in spring water,
drained

FOR THE DRESSING
4 tbsp fat free vinaigrette
1 tsp runny honey
juice of 1 lemon
1 tbsp wholegrain mustard
salt and freshly ground black pepper

TO SERVE
4 eggs, boiled to your liking (optional)

For a delicious variation on this summery French salad use cooked peeled prawns instead of the tuna.

Blanch the green beans in a large saucepan of lightly salted boiling water for 2–3 minutes, drain and refresh under cold running water. Drain and transfer to a large mixing bowl with the lettuce, cherry tomatoes and red onion.

Break the tuna into bite-sized pieces and add to the salad ingredients.

Make the dressing by whisking together all the ingredients, seasoning well. Pour over the tuna salad. Toss gently to mix and divide the salad between four plates. Garnish each serving with a halved boiled egg, if desired, and serve immediately.

Coq au vin

This popular dish originates in Provence, and with its bacon and button mushrooms in addition to the chicken it makes for hearty winter entertaining.

SERVES 4

EASY

Syns per serving
Extra Easy: 1½
Original: 1½
Green: 15

Preparation time 20 minutes
Cooking time about 40 minutes

low calorie cooking spray
12 lean bacon rashers, cut into large bite-sized pieces
12 baby onions, peeled but left whole
4 garlic cloves, peeled and crushed
400g/14oz baby button mushrooms
2 celery sticks, cut into 2cm/¾in pieces
2 carrots, peeled and cut into 2cm/¾in dice
1 thyme sprig
1 bay leaf
180ml/6fl oz red wine (Burgundy or Bordeaux)
800ml/28fl oz chicken stock
2 tbsp balsamic vinegar
12 skinless chicken thighs or drumsticks or 4 skinless chicken breast fillets
4–6 tbsp finely chopped flat-leaf parsley
salt and freshly ground black pepper

TO SERVE
a crisp green salad or green beans

Place a heavy-based flameproof casserole dish over a medium heat, spray with low calorie cooking spray and add the bacon and onions. Stir-fry until just browned; then stir in the garlic, mushrooms, celery and carrots. Turn up the heat to high and add the thyme, bay leaf, red wine, stock and vinegar.

Add the chicken and bring the mixture to the boil, then lower the heat and simmer gently for about 25 minutes or until the chicken is tender and cooked through.

For a thicker sauce, remove the chicken once it is cooked and keep warm. Cook the sauce over a high heat for a few minutes until the volume of liquid has reduced. Return the chicken to the pan.

Stir in the parsley, season well and serve with a crisp green salad or green beans.

Canard à l'orange

SERVES 4

WORTH THE EFFORT ❄

Syns per serving
Extra Easy: ½
Original: ½
Green: 14

Preparation time 10 minutes
Cooking time about 30 minutes

In this classic French dish, the rich flavour of the duck is complemented by the citrusy sweetness of the orange in the sauce.

FOR THE SAUCE
½ tbsp artificial sweetener
60ml/2fl oz white wine vinegar
juice and finely sliced zest of 1 orange
360ml/12fl oz chicken stock

FOR THE DUCK
4 skinless duck breasts, all visible fat removed
salt and freshly ground black pepper
2 garlic cloves, peeled and crushed
175g/6oz baby spinach leaves

To make the sauce, put the sweetener and vinegar into a medium-sized saucepan, bring to the boil and reduce until the liquid begins to caramelise. Add the orange juice, reduce down to one-third and add the stock. Reduce the heat and leave to simmer for 15–20 minutes. Add half the orange zest to the orange sauce and simmer for a further 2–3 minutes. Remove from the heat and keep warm.

Meanwhile, preheat the oven to 200°C/Gas 6. Score the skinned side of each duck breast with a diamond pattern and season.

Heat a large non-stick frying pan over a high heat and add the duck breasts, skinned sides down. Cook until lightly browned, turn the breasts over and cook for a further 30 seconds. Transfer to the oven and cook for 4–5 minutes, depending on size. When the breasts are cooked, remove them from the oven and leave to rest – skinned sides up.

Place the garlic and spinach in a saucepan with 60ml/2fl oz of water. Cook briefly over a medium–high heat until the spinach has wilted, then season to taste.

To serve, place a portion of drained spinach on each of four plates, cut each duck breast into slices and fan evenly across the spinach. Pour the sauce around the plate and garnish with the remaining orange zest.

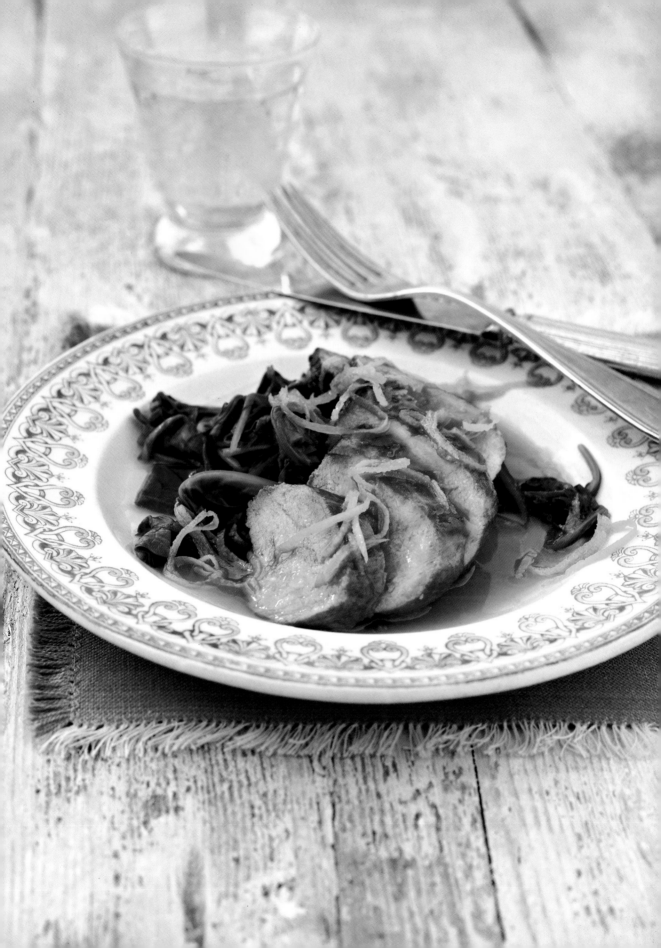

Basque-style chicken

SERVES 4

EASY ✳

Syns per serving
Extra Easy: ½
Original: ½
Green: 21

Preparation time 20 minutes
Cooking time just over an hour

salt and freshly ground black pepper
1.5kg/3lb 6oz chicken, skinned and
jointed into 8 pieces
1 large red pepper, deseeded
and thinly sliced
1 yellow pepper, deseeded
and thinly sliced
4–6 shallots, peeled and halved
4–6 garlic cloves, peeled and finely
chopped
600ml/1 pint chicken stock
100ml/3½fl oz passata
1 tsp sweet smoked paprika
8 black olives (optional)
1 lemon, thinly sliced
2 tbsp chopped tarragon
chopped flat-leaf parsley

The delicious combination of chicken, olives and peppers is typical of all the regions around the western Mediterranean, but this French version, with the addition of a hint of smoked paprika, beats the lot.

Season the chicken pieces well and place in a large flameproof casserole dish with the peppers, shallots and garlic. Add the stock, passata and paprika.

Place over a medium heat and as soon as everything reaches simmering point lower the heat to a gentle simmer. Scatter the olives, if using, and the lemon slices among the chicken pieces and sprinkle the tarragon over the top.

Cover with a tight-fitting lid and cook over the gentlest possible heat for 50 minutes–1 hour or until the chicken is cooked through.

Remove from the heat and scatter with chopped parsley just before serving.

Boeuf bourguignon

SERVES 4

EASY ✽

Syns per serving
Extra Easy: 1
Original: 1
Green: 13½

Preparation time 15 minutes
Cooking time 2½ hours

low calorie cooking spray
800g/1lb 12oz lean stewing beef, cut
into bite-sized pieces
2 garlic cloves, peeled and crushed
12 large shallots, peeled and halved
3 carrots, peeled and roughly chopped
200g/7oz baby button mushrooms
1 thyme sprig
600ml/1 pint beef stock
100ml/3½fl oz red wine
salt and freshly ground black pepper
2 tsp dried herbes de Provence
chopped flat-leaf parsley

This dish is a well-known traditional French recipe. It is essentially a stew prepared with beef braised in beef stock and a robust red wine, such as a good Burgundy.

Preheat the oven to 160°C/Gas 3. Spray a large non-stick frying pan with low calorie cooking spray and place over a medium heat. Add the beef and stir-fry until brown on all sides.

Transfer to a medium casserole dish with the garlic, shallots, carrots, mushrooms, thyme, stock and wine. Season well and add the dried herbs.

Cover tightly and cook in the oven for 2½ hours or until the beef is tender and cooked through. Remove from the oven and sprinkle with chopped parsley before serving.

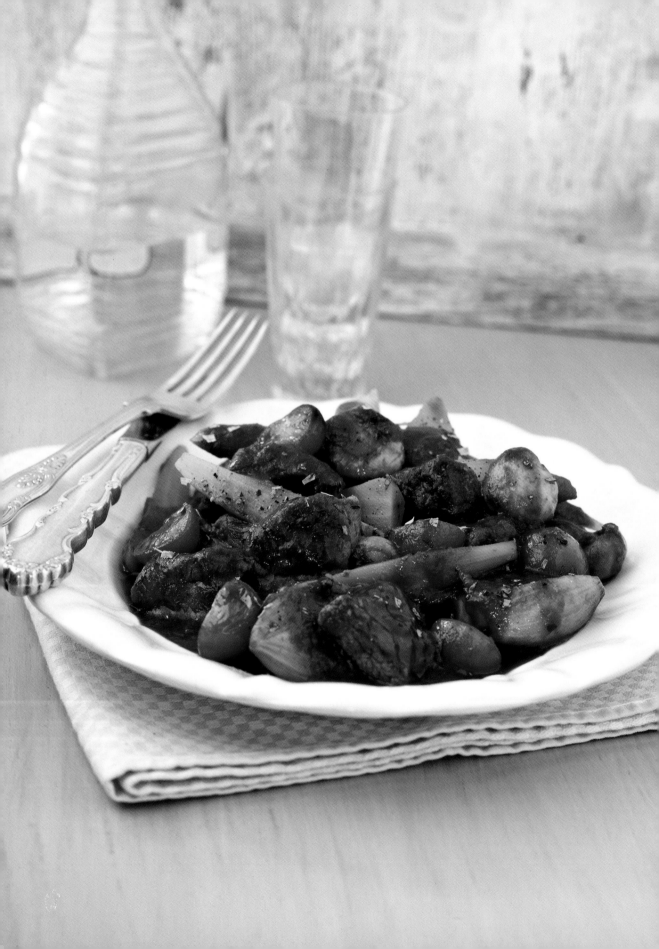

Navarin of lamb

This wonderfully flavoured casserole uses tender lamb cooked in a rich tomato sauce with a variety of vegetables.

SERVES 4

EASY ✳

Syns per serving
Extra Easy: Free
Original: 3
Green: 19½

Preparation time 20 minutes
Cooking time just under 2 hours

low calorie cooking spray
1kg/2lb 4oz lean neck or shoulder of lamb, cut into 2.5cm/1in cubes
900ml/1½ pints lamb or beef stock
400g can chopped tomatoes
salt and freshly ground black pepper
1 bouquet garni
6 shallots, peeled and halved
12 baby carrots, peeled and cut in half lengthways
12 baby parsnips, peeled and cut in half lengthways
200g/7oz cherry tomatoes, halved
200g/7oz baby button mushrooms

TO SERVE
chopped flat-leaf parsley

Spray a large non-stick frying pan with low calorie cooking spray and place over a medium heat. Add the lamb and fry on all sides until lightly browned.

Stir in the stock and tomatoes and bring to the boil. Season well and add the bouquet garni. Cover, reduce the heat and simmer for about 1 hour.

Remove the bouquet garni and add the shallots, carrots and parsnips and continue cooking for a further 30 minutes. Finally, add the cherry tomatoes and mushrooms and continue cooking for 10–12 minutes, until tender.

Serve on a warmed serving dish, garnished with chopped parsley.

Crêpes Suzette

SERVES 4

EASY Ⓥ

Syns per serving
Extra Easy: 6
Original: 6
Green: 6

Preparation time 20 minutes
Cooking time 15–20 minutes

FOR THE SAUCE
juice of 2 oranges
2–3 tbsp artificial sweetener

FOR THE CRÊPES
110g/4oz wholemeal flour
3 tbsp artificial sweetener
a pinch of salt
2 large eggs, beaten
300ml/½ pint skimmed milk
2 tbsp orange juice
1 tbsp finely grated orange zest
2–3 drops vanilla extract
low calorie cooking spray

TO SERVE
fresh orange segments
fat free natural fromage frais

In this version of a French classic we've omitted the flambéed liqueur but it's so delicious, we don't think you'll notice it's not there.

First make the sauce by placing the orange juice and sweetener in a small saucepan. Stir over a gentle heat until the sweetener has dissolved. Remove from the heat and set aside.

For the crêpes, sift the flour, sweetener and salt into a bowl or measuring jug. Mix in the eggs, milk, orange juice and zest and vanilla extract and whisk until smooth.

Spray a 15cm/6in non-stick frying pan with low calorie cooking spray and place over a high heat. Pour approximately one-eighth of the batter into the pan, tilting the pan to spread the batter. Cook for 1–2 minutes or until the underside is lightly browned, then carefully flip over and cook for a further 1–2 minutes. Remove the crêpe, fold into quarters and keep warm while you cook the remaining seven crêpes.

Divide the folded crêpes between four warmed plates, drizzle with the orange sauce and serve with fresh orange segments and a dollop of fromage frais.

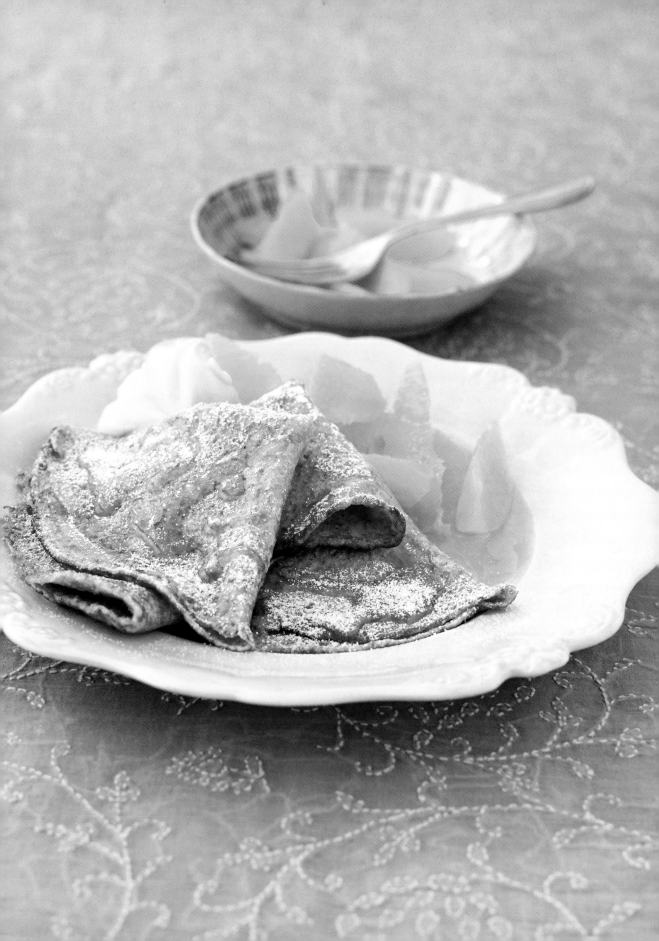

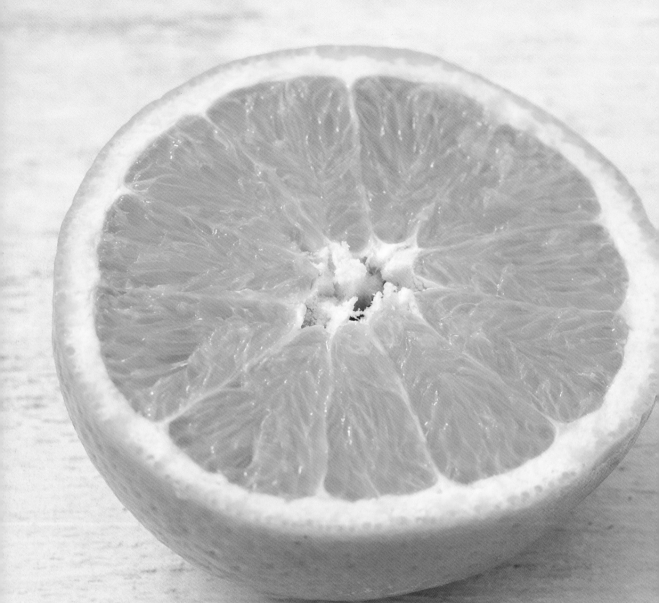

Spain

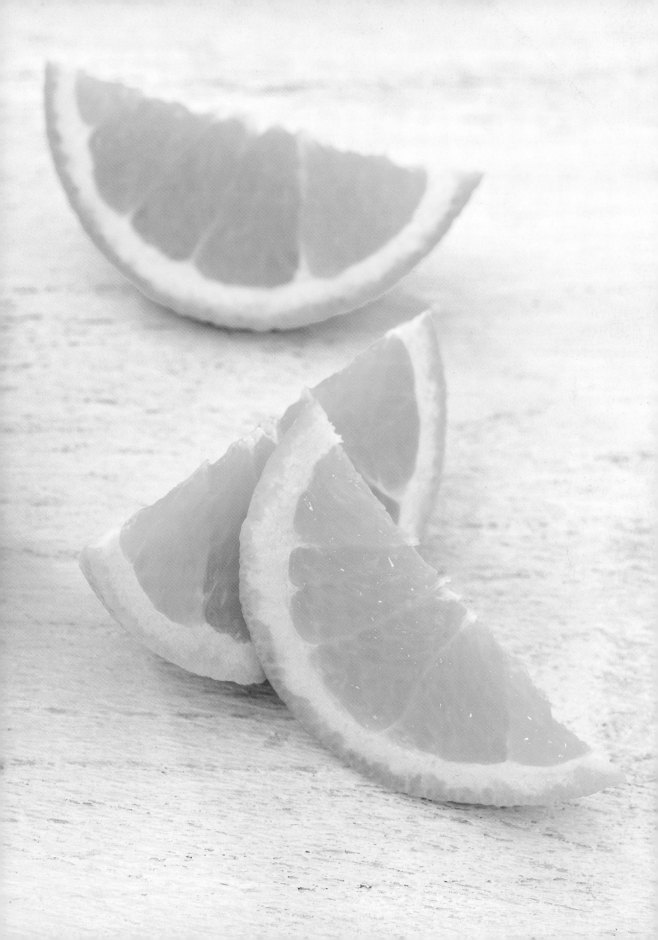

Gazpacho

SERVES 4–6

EASY (V) (❄)

Syns per serving
Extra Easy: Free
Original: Free
Green: Free

Preparation time under 20 minutes
plus chilling time

7–8 large plum or vine tomatoes
1 bottled roasted red pepper, drained
and roughly chopped
2 garlic cloves, peeled and crushed
¼ tsp artificial sweetener (optional)
2–3 tbsp red wine vinegar
a few drops of Tabasco sauce
salt and freshly ground black pepper

TO SERVE
4 tbsp finely diced cucumber
3 tbsp finely diced red pepper

Use the ripest plum or vine tomatoes to maximize the flavour of this wonderful chilled, summery soup.

To remove the skins from the tomatoes, score a cross in the base of each tomato and place in a bowl of boiling water for 10–15 seconds. Drain and plunge into cold water then peel off the skins. Cut the tomatoes in half and deseed them. Roughly chop the flesh and place in a food processor.

Add the roasted red pepper, garlic, sweetener if using, vinegar and Tabasco sauce and process until smooth, adding up to 300ml/11fl oz of chilled water if you want a thinner consistency. Season and chill for 3–4 hours or overnight if time permits.

To serve, pour the gazpacho into chilled glasses and top with a little of the garnishes.

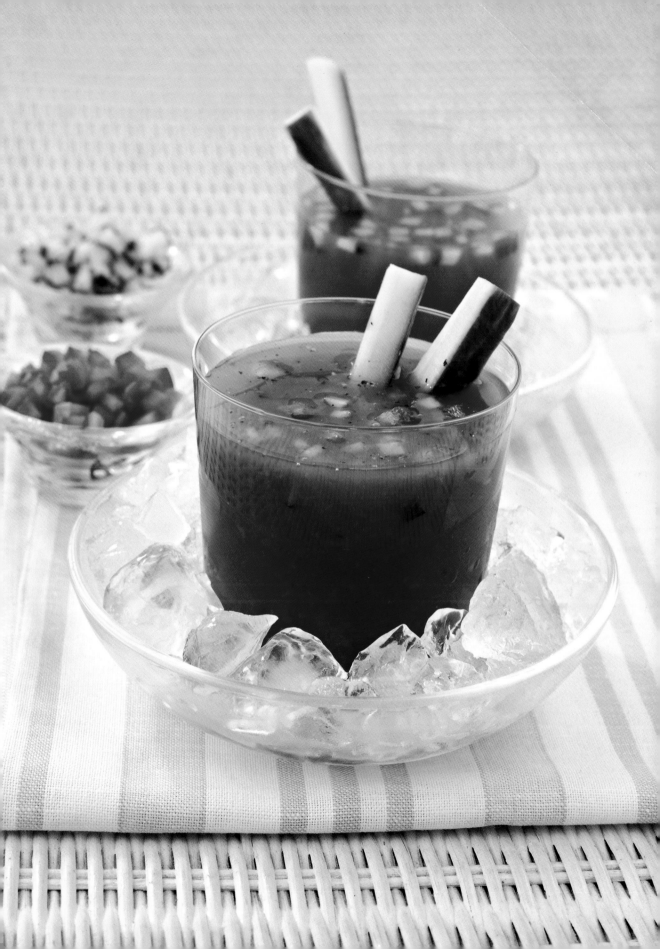

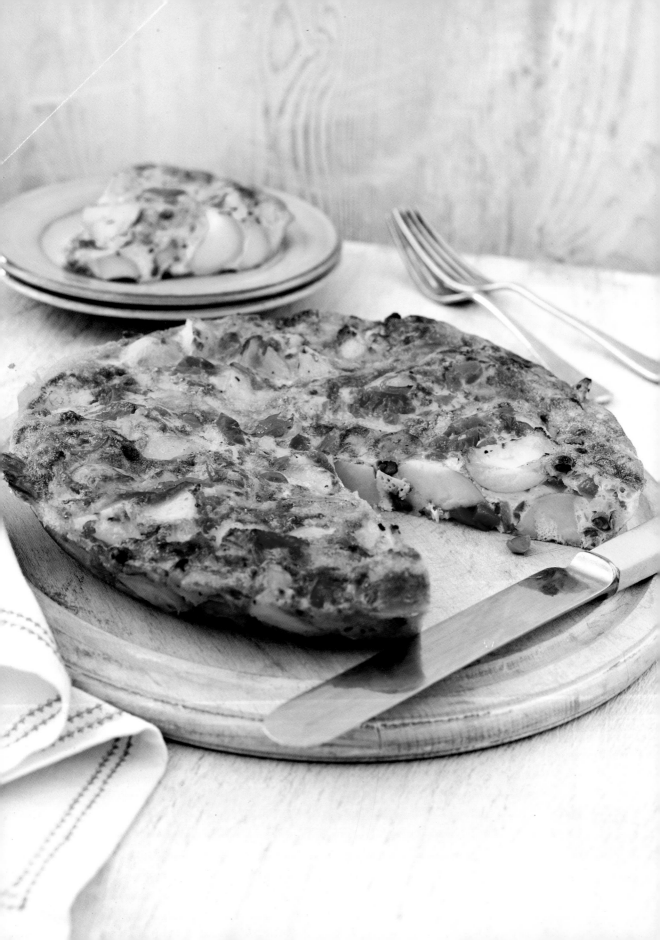

Spanish onion, pepper, pea and potato tortilla

SERVES 4–6

EASY Ⓥ ❋

Syns per serving
Extra Easy: Free
Green: Free
Original: 4

Preparation time 15 minutes
Cooking time 30–35 minutes

250g/9oz potatoes, peeled and cut into 1cm/½in cubes
low calorie cooking spray
3 onions, peeled and finely sliced
200g/7oz bottled roasted red peppers, drained and roughly chopped
200g/7oz frozen peas, thawed
2 garlic cloves, peeled and finely chopped
5 eggs
salt and freshly ground black pepper

Tortillas like this one can be made up to a day in advance and stored in the fridge until you are ready to serve it. Just bring it back to room temperature before serving.

Parboil the potatoes in a large saucepan of lightly salted boiling water for 5–6 minutes. Drain thoroughly.

Spray a 20–23cm/8–9in non-stick frying pan with low calorie cooking spray and place over a medium heat. Add the onions, peppers, peas and drained potatoes, and fry gently over a medium heat for 12–15 minutes or until the vegetables have softened, but not coloured, turning and stirring often. Add the garlic and stir to mix well.

Preheat the grill to medium–hot.

In a bowl, beat the eggs lightly and season well. Pour this mixture into the frying pan, shaking the pan so that the egg and vegetables are evenly spread. Cook gently for 8–10 minutes or until the tortilla is set at the bottom.

Place the frying pan under the grill and cook for 5–6 minutes or until the top is set and golden. Remove from the grill and allow to cool for 5–6 minutes. Carefully transfer to a board and cut into wedges. Serve warm or at room temperature.

Huevos rellenos

SERVES 4

WORTH THE EFFORT

Syns per serving
Extra Easy: ½
Original: ½
Green: 2

Preparation time 20–30 minutes

Stuffed eggs are popular the world over and are loved by children and adults alike. These are quick and easy to prepare. You can vary the fish used in this recipe by using flaked salmon if desired.

4 hard-boiled eggs
100g/3½oz canned tuna in spring water, drained
2 tbsp extra light mayonnaise
1 tbsp passata
a pinch of sweet pimentón or paprika
salt and freshly ground black pepper

TO SERVE
1 tbsp finely chopped black olives
1 tbsp finely chopped bottled roasted red pepper
1 tbsp finely chopped flat-leaf parsley

Halve the boiled eggs lengthways and carefully scoop out the yolks into a bowl. Place the egg whites, cut sides up on a serving plate and set aside.

Flake the tuna and add to the yolks with the mayonnaise, passata and pimentón or paprika. Season well and stir to mix until thoroughly combined.

Spoon the fish mixture carefully into the egg whites using a teaspoon. Lightly cover and chill until ready to serve.

Before serving, garnish with the black olives and red pepper and sprinkle over some parsley.

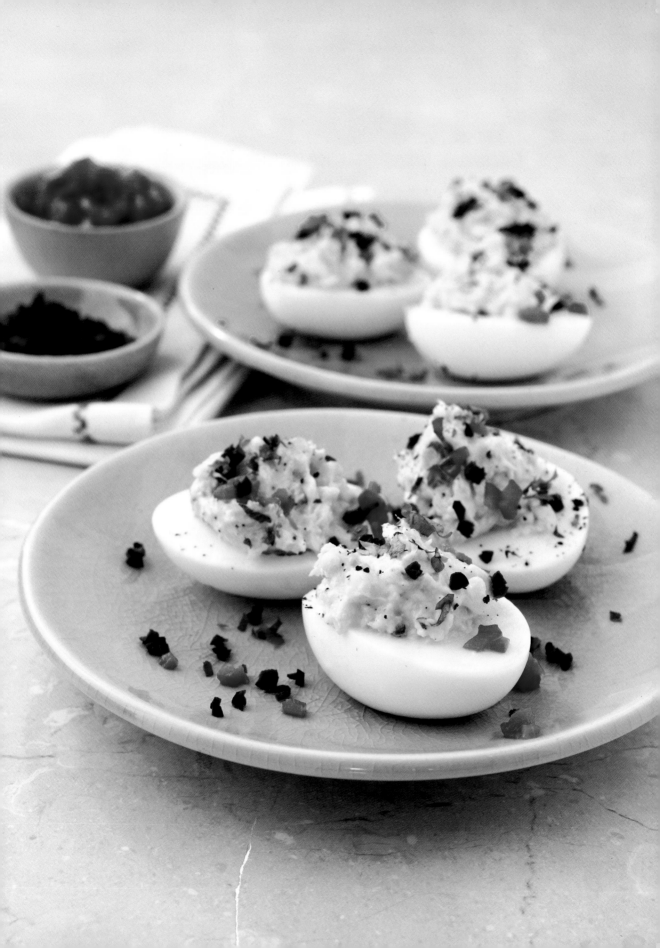

Judías verdes

SERVES 4

EASY (V) (✳)

Syns per serving
Extra Easy: Free
Original: Free
Green: Free

Preparation time 10 minutes
Cooking time about 15 minutes

1 tbsp white wine vinegar
400g/14oz green beans, trimmed
low calorie cooking spray
1 small onion, peeled and finely diced
2 garlic cloves, peeled and finely diced
salt and freshly ground black pepper

Lightly cooked and fried beans are a popular dish in Spain. For a change, you can substitute mangetout or sugar snap peas for the green beans.

Bring a large saucepan of water to the boil. Add the vinegar and beans, bring back to the boil and cook for 3–4 minutes. Drain, refresh the beans in cold water and drain again. Pat the beans dry with kitchen paper.

Spray a large non-stick frying pan with low calorie cooking spray and place over a medium heat. Add the onion and beans and sauté for 3–4 minutes, then add the garlic and sauté for 1 more minute.

Season well, cover the pan and reduce the heat to very low. Cook for a further 5–6 minutes until the beans are cooked, then remove from the heat and serve immediately.

Patatas bravas

SERVES 4

WORTH THE EFFORT (V) (❄)

Syns per serving
Extra Easy: Free
Green: Free
Original: 7½

Preparation time 20 minutes
Cooking time 30–35 minutes

800g/1lb 12oz potatoes, peeled
and cut into bite-sized pieces
low calorie cooking spray
salt and freshly ground black pepper
400g can chopped tomatoes
1 small red onion, peeled
and finely chopped
2 garlic cloves, peeled
and finely chopped
3 tsp sweet pimentón or paprika
1 bay leaf

TO SERVE
finely chopped flat-leaf parsley

This Spanish tapas snack of potatoes with a tomato sauce can be found in tapas bars across Spain. It is equally successful served as a main course with a side salad or green vegetables.

Preheat the oven to 220°C/Gas 7 and line a baking sheet with baking parchment. Parboil the potatoes in a large saucepan of lightly salted water for 5–6 minutes. Drain the potatoes thoroughly, transfer to the baking sheet and spray with low calorie cooking spray. Season well and roast in the oven for 15–20 minutes, until lightly browned.

While the potatoes are roasting, place the tomatoes, red onion and garlic in a saucepan and place over a medium heat. Cook for 10–15 minutes, then add the pimentón or paprika and bay leaf. Continue to stir and cook for 5–10 minutes, until the tomatoes are softened.

Remove the potatoes to a warmed serving dish and pour over the tomato sauce. Toss to mix well, garnish with parsley and serve.

Escalivada

WORTH THE EFFORT Ⓥ ❋

Syns per serving
Extra Easy: 1½
Original: 1½
Green: 1½

Preparation time 15 minutes
Cooking time 30 minutes

1 large aubergine
1 red pepper
1 yellow pepper
1 large Spanish onion, unpeeled
2 courgettes
4 tomatoes
4 garlic cloves, unpeeled
1 tbsp olive oil
1 tbsp red wine vinegar
or sherry vinegar
juice of ½ lemon
salt and freshly ground black pepper
1 tbsp chopped flat-leaf parsley

This vegetable salad can be eaten warm or cold and is a wonderful accompaniment for grilled fish, chicken or lamb. The vegetables can be cooked on a barbecue; over hot coals for a more smoky flavour.

Preheat the oven to 180°C/Gas 4. Put the aubergine, peppers, onion, courgettes and tomatoes in an ovenproof baking dish. Tuck the garlic cloves in between them and sprinkle the oil over the top. Roast in the oven for about 30 minutes until the vegetables are tender and slightly charred.

Remove from the oven and cut the aubergine into strips. Peel and deseed the peppers, and cut the flesh into strips. Peel the onion and cut into wedges. Trim the courgettes and slice thinly. Transfer to a serving dish.

Peel the tomatoes and garlic cloves and mash them together with any oil left in the baking dish, and the vinegar and lemon juice. Pour over the roasted vegetables, season and sprinkle with chopped parsley. Leave to cool before serving, but do not chill – this is best served at room temperature.

Zarzuela

The name 'zarzuela' actually means a 'light opera' in Spain, but it has also been given to this style of lively, spicy fish stew. You can use any kind of mixed seafood and shellfish in this recipe.

SERVES 4

WORTH THE EFFORT ❄ (only if fish are fresh)

Syns per serving
Extra Easy: Free
Original: Free
Green: 13

Preparation time 25 minutes
Cooking time under 30 minutes

low calorie cooking spray
12 raw tiger prawns in their shells
1 onion, peeled and finely chopped
4 garlic cloves, peeled and crushed
4 medium tomatoes, chopped
1 bay leaf
a large pinch of saffron threads
1 tsp sweet pimentón or paprika
1 dried red chilli, chopped
270ml/9fl oz fish stock
400g/14oz firm white fish fillets (cod, halibut), cut into bite-sized pieces
4 small squid, cleaned and sliced
12 clams, scrubbed
8 mussels, scrubbed
3 tbsp finely chopped flat-leaf parsley
salt and freshly ground black pepper

Spray a large non-stick frying pan with low calorie cooking spray, add the prawns and sauté over a medium heat until they start to turn pink. Remove with a slotted spoon onto a plate and set aside.

Add the onion and half of the garlic cloves to the frying pan and cook gently for 10 minutes, until the onion has softened. Add the tomatoes, bay leaf, saffron, pimentón or paprika, dried chilli and stock. Bring to the boil and then add the fish and squid. Cook for 5 minutes, add the clams and mussels and cook for a further 5–8 minutes or until they open, discard any mussels that remain closed.

Add the remaining garlic and the parsley. Season well and return the prawns with any juices back to the pan. Stir to mix thoroughly and then ladle into shallow soup plates and eat immediately.

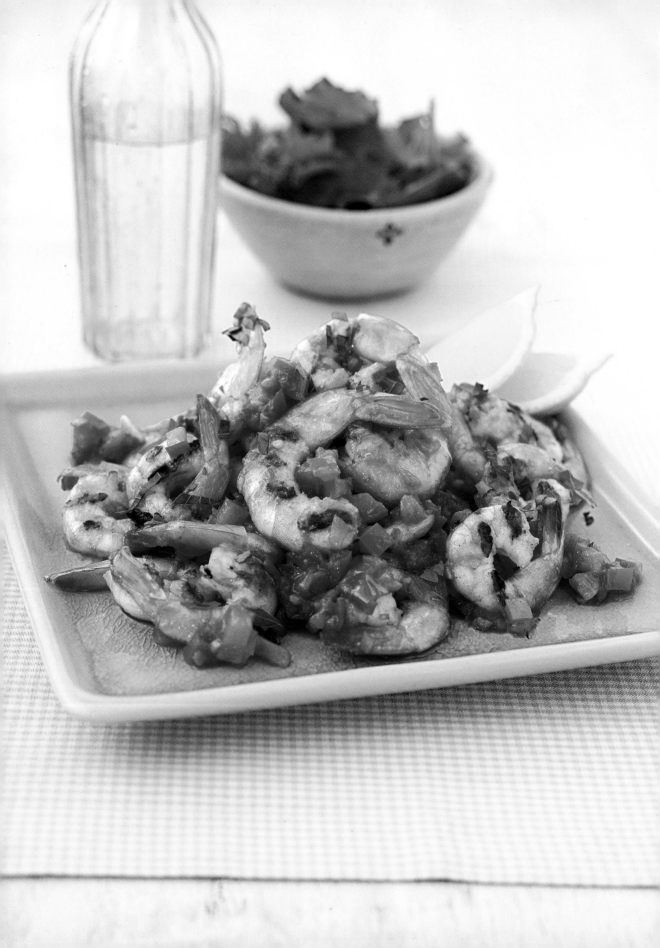

Gambas con romesco

SERVES 4

EASY ✳ (only if prawns are fresh)

Syns per serving
Extra Easy: Free
Original: Free
Green: 4½

Preparation time 20 minutes
Cooking time about 10 minutes

Grilled prawns are served with the classic, spicy tomato sauce from Catalonia.

low calorie cooking spray
1 large red pepper, deseeded
and chopped
1 dried red chilli, chopped
250g/9oz tomatoes, chopped
4 garlic cloves, peeled and crushed
90ml/3fl oz red wine vinegar
salt and freshly ground black pepper
20 large raw tiger prawns, peeled but
with tails left on

TO SERVE
chopped flat-leaf parsley

Spray a large non-stick frying pan with low calorie cooking spray and place over a medium heat. Add the pepper, chilli, tomatoes and garlic to the pan and sauté for 5–6 minutes. Remove from the heat and allow to cool. Stir in the vinegar and check the seasoning.

Meanwhile, preheat the grill to hot and place the prawns on a grill rack. Lightly spray with low calorie cooking spray, place under the grill and cook for 2–3 minutes on each side or until they turn pink and are just cooked through. Toss the prawns in the sauce, garnish with chopped parsley and eat immediately.

Valencian paella

SERVES 6

EASY ✳ (only if shellfish are fresh)

Syns per serving
Extra Easy: Free
Green: 5½
Original: 21

Preparation time 25–30 minutes
Cooking time under an hour

200g/7oz skinless and boneless
chicken thighs, cut into
bite-sized pieces
salt and freshly ground black pepper
low calorie cooking spray
2 medium onions, peeled
and finely chopped
4 garlic cloves, peeled and chopped
2 red peppers, deseeded and chopped
680g/1lb 8oz dried paella rice
3 tbsp finely chopped flat-leaf parsley
1 bay leaf
a large pinch of saffron threads
1.5 litres/2½ pints chicken stock
100g/3½oz shelled broad beans
12 large raw tiger prawns,
peeled but with tails left on
12 mussels, cleaned and beards
removed

TO SERVE
chopped flat-leaf parsley
lemon wedges (optional)

The famous combination of chicken, prawns and shellfish, flavoured with saffron and garlic, makes a perfect spread for entertaining, especially when eating al fresco.

Pat the chicken pieces dry with kitchen paper and season well. Spray a paella pan or a wide non-stick frying pan with low calorie cooking spray and place over a medium heat. Sauté the chicken pieces until golden. Lift out with a slotted spoon and keep warm.

Add the onions, garlic and red peppers to the pan and sauté for 4–5 minutes. Return the chicken to the pan and stir in the rice, parsley, bay leaf and saffron. Stir in the stock and broad beans, bring to a simmer and cook, uncovered, over a gentle heat for 12–15 minutes. Add the prawns and mussels.

Cover tightly, turn the heat to very low and allow to cook for another 12–15 minutes or until the rice is tender, the prawns are cooked and the mussels have opened up and all the liquid is absorbed. Remove from the heat and discard any mussels that remain closed. Let the paella stand covered for 10 minutes. Garnish with chopped parsley and lemon wedges, if using, and serve.

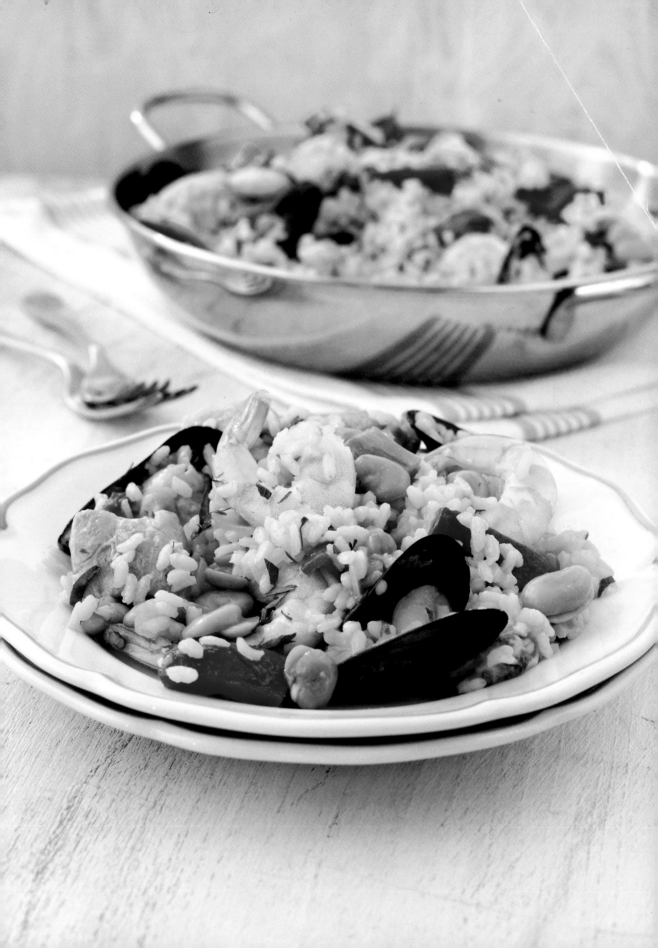

Vieras de vigo

SERVES 4

EASY

Syns per serving
Extra Easy: 2
Original: 2
Green: 4

Preparation time 15 minutes
Cooking time 6–8 minutes

12 medium scallops, roughly chopped
1 garlic clove, peeled and very finely chopped
1 tbsp very finely chopped shallot
2 tbsp very finely chopped tomato
¼ tsp finely grated lemon zest
1 tbsp lemon juice
2 tbsp very finely chopped flat-leaf parsley
salt and freshly ground black pepper
3 tbsp fresh wholemeal breadcrumbs

For an impressive presentation, ask your fishmonger to give you the scallop shells so that you can use them when grilling the scallop mixture.

Put the scallops in a bowl and add the garlic, shallots, tomato, lemon zest and juice and parsley. Season well and mix to combine.

Preheat the grill to medium–hot. Divide the scallop mixture between eight scallop shells and sprinkle over the breadcrumbs. Place the filled shells under the grill for 6–8 minutes or until lightly golden and just cooked through. Serve immediately.

Pollo al chilindrón

SERVES 4

EASY ❄

Syns per serving
Extra Easy: Free
Original: Free
Green: 10½

Preparation time 20 minutes
Cooking time just over 1½ hours

low calorie cooking spray
1kg/2lb 4oz skinless chicken thighs
4 garlic cloves, peeled and crushed
1 onion, peeled and finely chopped
4 lean bacon rashers, diced
3 red peppers, deseeded and thinly
sliced
400g can chopped tomatoes
1 thyme sprig
1 bay leaf
salt and freshly ground black pepper

TO SERVE
chopped flat-leaf parsley

For an interesting variation on this rich red pepper and tomato one-pot dish, you could replace the chicken with cubed veal or beef.

Spray a large non-stick saucepan with low calorie cooking spray and place over a medium heat. Add the chicken, garlic and onion and stir-fry for 4–5 minutes.

Add the bacon and peppers and stir-fry for 1–2 minutes and then add the tomatoes, thyme and bay leaf. Bring to the boil, cover tightly and reduce the heat to very low. Cook for about 1½ hours, until the chicken is meltingly tender.

Season well, garnish with chopped parsley and serve immediately.

Albóndigas

These spiced meatballs – tossed in a flavoured tomato sauce – are a tapas favourite all around Spain.

SERVES 4

WORTH THE EFFORT ❋

Syns per serving
Extra Easy: Free
Original: Free
Green: 5

Preparation time 20 minutes plus chilling time
Cooking time about 45 minutes

300g/11oz extra lean minced pork
3 garlic cloves, peeled and crushed
1 tsp ground cumin
1 tsp ground coriander
1 tsp ground nutmeg
1 tsp ground cinnamon
salt and freshly ground black pepper
low calorie cooking spray

FOR THE SAUCE
1 small onion, peeled and finely chopped
1 garlic clove, peeled and crushed
400g can chopped tomatoes
1 tsp sweet pimentón or paprika

Place the pork, garlic and spices in a bowl and, using your hands, mix until thoroughly combined. Season well. Cover and chill in the fridge for 1 hour to allow the flavours to develop.

Meanwhile, make the sauce by placing the onion, garlic, tomatoes and sweet pimentón or paprika in a large heavy-based saucepan, stir and cook over a medium heat for 5–6 minutes. Reduce the heat, cover and simmer gently for 25–30 minutes, stirring occasionally.

To make the meatballs: make small walnut shaped balls from the mince mixture. Spray a large non-stick frying pan with low calorie cooking spray and stir-fry half the meatballs over a medium heat for 2–3 minutes until browned. Drain on kitchen paper and repeat with the remaining meatballs.

Place the sauce mixture over a medium heat and add the meatballs. Stir to coat evenly and simmer gently for 5–6 minutes Serve hot.

Cochifrito

SERVES 4

EASY ❄

Syns per serving
Extra Easy: Free
Original: Free
Green: 17½

Preparation time 10 minutes
Cooking time about 1 hour 40 minutes

900g/2lb lean boneless lamb, cut into
bite-sized pieces
salt and freshly ground black pepper
low calorie cooking spray
4 garlic cloves, peeled and crushed
1 onion, peeled and finely chopped
1 tbsp sweet pimentón or paprika
3 tbsp lemon juice
4 tbsp finely chopped flat-leaf parsley
100ml/3½fl oz lamb stock

This delicious stew hails from the Aragon region in north-eastern Spain. The delicate flavour of the lamb is enhanced by lemon, garlic and parsley.

Season the lamb well with salt and pepper. Spray a large non-stick frying pan with low calorie cooking spray and place over a high heat. Add the lamb and brown all over for 6–8 minutes.

Transfer to a heavy-based casserole dish and add the garlic, onion, pimentón or paprika, lemon juice, parsley and stock. Cover tightly and cook over a low heat for 1½ hours or until the lamb is meltingly tender. Serve immediately.

Spanish orange cake

SERVES 12

EASY (V)

Syns per serving
Extra Easy: 4
Original: 4
Green: 4

Preparation time 30 minutes
Cooking time about 30 minutes

FOR THE CAKE
4 eggs, separated
50g/2oz golden caster sugar
5 tbsp artificial sweetener
150g/5oz self-raising flour
1 tsp baking powder
2 tbsp finely grated orange zest
juice of 2 oranges

FOR THE SYRUP
zest of 2 oranges, finely grated into
long strips
juice of 2 oranges
1 tbsp arrowroot
4 tbsp Splenda Brown Sugar Blend

TO SERVE
fresh raspberries
long strips of grated orange zest

Spain is famous for its oranges. Here they are used in this moist cake, which can be made up to two days in advance, if stored in an air-tight container.

Preheat the oven to 190°C/Gas 5. Line a 20cm/8in cake tin with non-stick baking parchment.

Place the egg yolks, caster sugar, sweetener, self-raising flour, baking powder and orange zest and juice in a bowl and whisk until thick and pale.

In a separate bowl, whisk the egg whites until softly peaked then fold them into the egg yolk mixture. Spoon this mixture into the prepared cake tin and cook in the oven for 25–30 minutes or until the cake is risen and firm to the touch. Leave to cool.

Meanwhile place all the syrup ingredients in a small saucepan with 90ml/3fl oz of water and bring to the boil, whisking constantly. When it starts to thicken, remove from the heat.

Drizzle the syrup over the cake and decorate with raspberries and grated orange zest. Cut into wedges to serve.

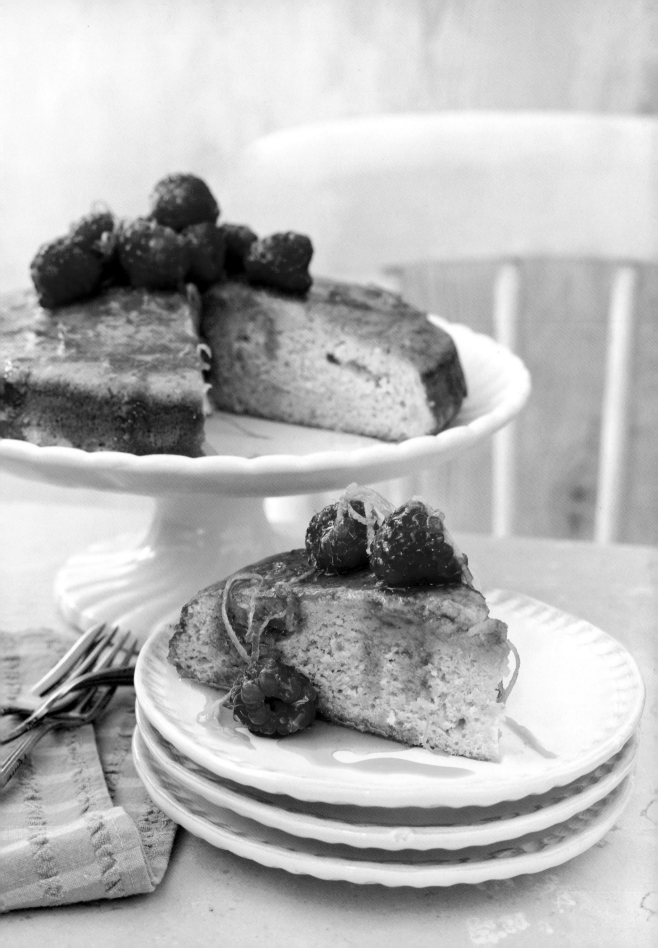

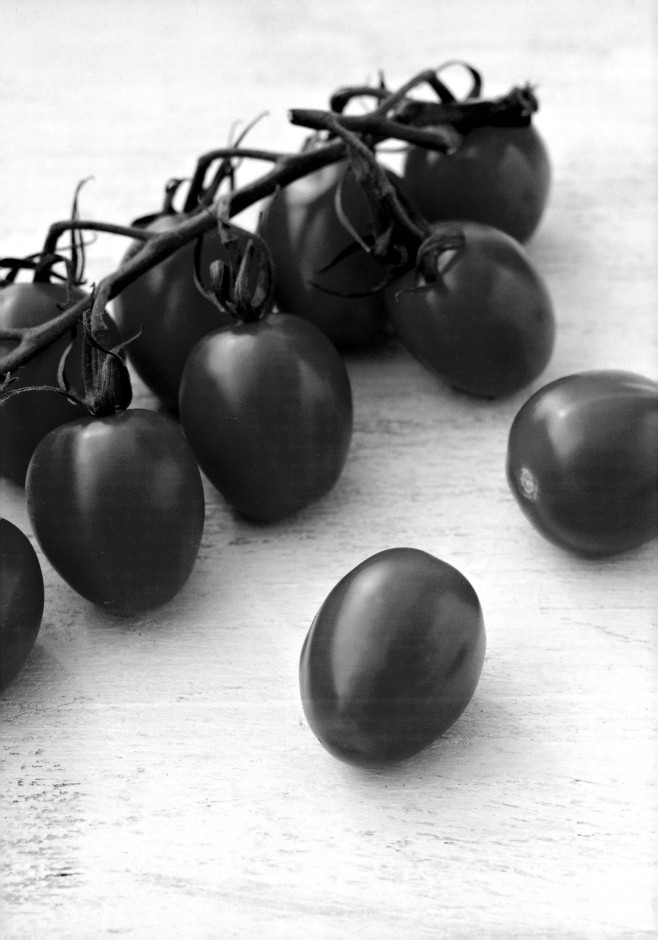

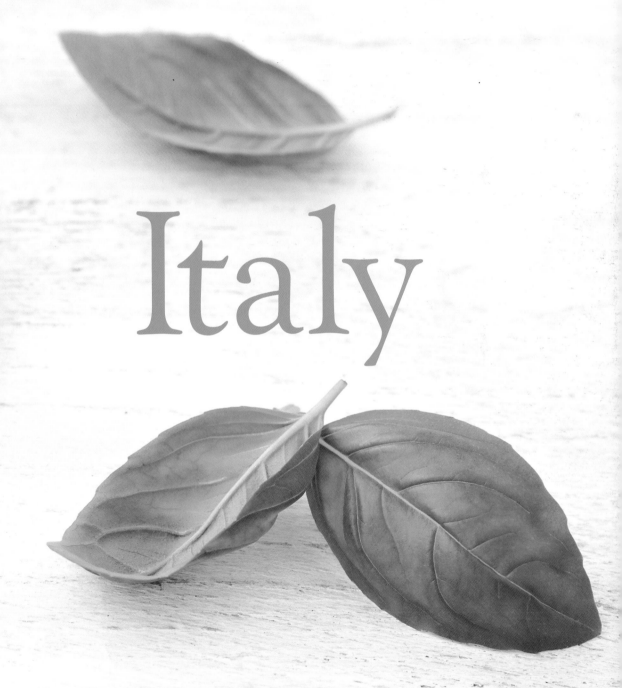

Italy

Tuscan bean and pasta soup

SERVES 4

EASY Ⓥ ❄

Syns per serving
Extra Easy: 3½
Green: 3½
Original: 11½

Preparation time 25 minutes plus
overnight soaking
Cooking time 1¼–1½ hours

175g/6oz dried cannellini beans
1 onion, peeled and chopped
1 leek, trimmed and chopped
2 carrots, peeled and chopped
1 celery stick, chopped
1 fennel bulb, trimmed and chopped
225g/8oz tomatoes,
skinned and chopped
2 garlic cloves, peeled and crushed
1.25 litres/2 pints vegetable stock
50g/2oz dried pasta shapes
450g/1lb greens or dark green cabbage,
trimmed and shredded
salt and freshly ground black pepper
2 tbsp chopped flat-leaf parsley
4 x 25g/1oz slices French bread
1–2 garlic cloves, peeled and left whole

TO SERVE
chopped chives

This robust Italian soup of cannellini beans and pasta shapes is warming and reviving on a cold winter's day. If you serve the soup without the garlic bread, it will be Free on Green and Extra Easy.

Soak the beans in cold water overnight. Drain them and rinse under cold running water.

Put the beans in a large saucepan with the onion, leek, carrots, celery, fennel, tomatoes, crushed garlic and stock and bring to the boil. Reduce the heat to a simmer and cook very gently for 1 hour.

Stir in the pasta and the greens or cabbage, and cook for 15–30 minutes, until the beans, pasta and vegetables are cooked and tender. Season to taste and stir in the parsley.

Just before serving, preheat the grill to hot. Rub the slices of French bread on both sides with the garlic and toast them under the grill, until golden brown. Ladle the soup into bowls, top each serving with a slice of garlic toast and sprinkle with chives.

Vegetable lasagne

Preparation time 15 minutes
Cooking time 50 minutes

1 red pepper, deseeded and cut into chunks
1 yellow pepper, deseeded and cut into chunks
1 red onion, peeled, thickly sliced and cubed
2 courgettes, thickly sliced
1 aubergine, cubed
1 garlic clove, peeled and crushed
1 tbsp mixed herbs
salt and freshly ground black pepper
1 tsp oil
500ml/18fl oz passata
8–10 pre-cooked lasagne sheets
2 tbsp grated Parmesan cheese

FOR THE WHITE SAUCE
2 tbsp cornflour
300ml/½ pint skimmed milk
150g/5oz fat free natural fromage frais
a pinch of freshly grated nutmeg

You don't have to use meat in a lasagne – roasted vegetables make a colourful and delicious alternative. The advantage of this pasta dish is that it can be assembled several hours ahead or even the day before and kept in the fridge until you are ready to cook and serve it.

Preheat the oven to 200°C/Gas 6. Put the peppers, onion, courgettes, aubergine and garlic on a baking sheet or in a large roasting tin. Sprinkle with the mixed herbs and seasoning and drizzle the oil over the vegetables.

Roast the vegetables in the oven for about 20 minutes, until they are tender and just starting to look charred around the edges. Remove from the oven, transfer to a bowl and mix with the passata. Turn down the oven temperature to 190°C/Gas 5.

Meanwhile, make the white sauce. In a cup, blend the cornflour with a little of the milk. Heat the remaining milk in a saucepan and bring to the boil. Turn down the heat. Stir in the cornflour mixture and cook for 1–2 minutes, stirring, until thick. Remove from the heat and beat in the fromage frais and nutmeg. Season to taste.

Put half of the roasted vegetables in a 20 x 30cm/8 x 12inch ovenproof dish. Cover with half the lasagne sheets and spread with a little of the white sauce. Top with the remaining vegetables then the lasagne sheets and finish with the sauce. Sprinkle with the Parmesan cheese and bake in the oven for about 25 minutes, until golden.

Baked cannelloni

SERVES 4

EASY Ⓥ ✳

Syns per serving
Extra Easy: 1
Green: 1
Original: 5

Preparation time 15 minutes
Cooking time 30 minutes

FOR THE FILLING
225g/8oz spinach, trimmed
225g/8oz fat free natural cottage
cheese
freshly grated nutmeg
1 egg yolk
salt and freshly ground black pepper

FOR THE CANNELLONI
8 dried cannelloni tubes
450ml/3/4 pint passata
1/2 tsp sugar
1 garlic clove, peeled and crushed
a handful of basil leaves, torn (optional)
2 tbsp grated Parmesan cheese
(optional)

This quick and easy version of the classic baked pasta dish is made with dried canneloni tubes, which you can buy in most supermarkets.

Preheat the oven to 200°C/Gas 6.

To make the filling, put the spinach in a saucepan with 2 tablespoons of water. Cover with a lid and cook very gently over a low heat for about 5 minutes, until the leaves have wilted and turned bright green. Drain in a colander, pressing down on top of the spinach with a saucer to squeeze out all the liquid.

Chop the spinach and mix with the cottage cheese, nutmeg, egg yolk and seasoning. Spoon the filling into the cannelloni tubes and arrange them in an ovenproof dish.

To make the sauce, mix together the passata, sugar and garlic, season to taste and pour over the cannelloni. Sprinkle with the basil leaves and Parmesan cheese, if using, and bake in the oven for about 25 minutes, until bubbling and golden brown.

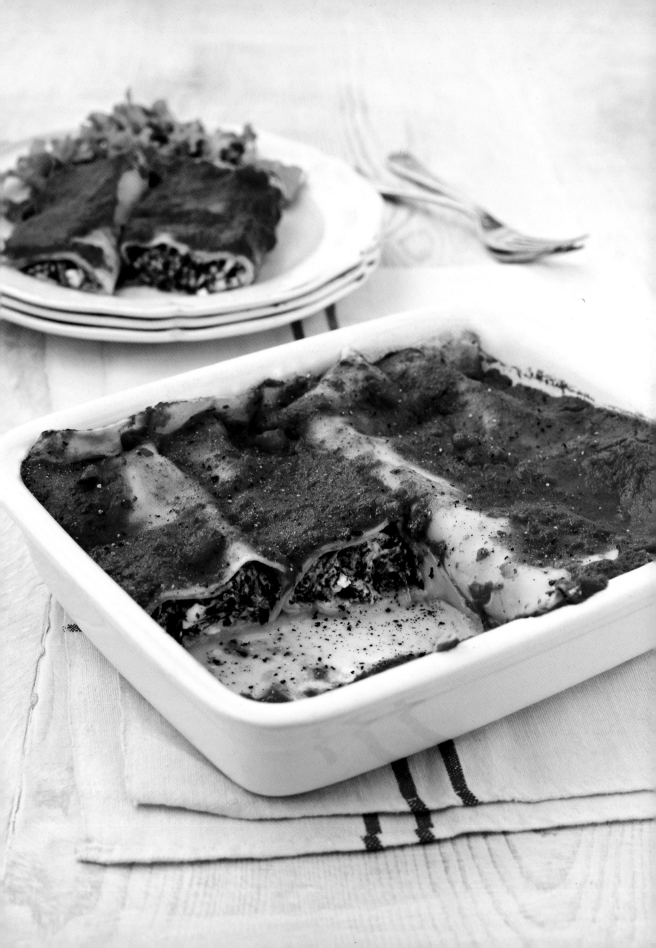

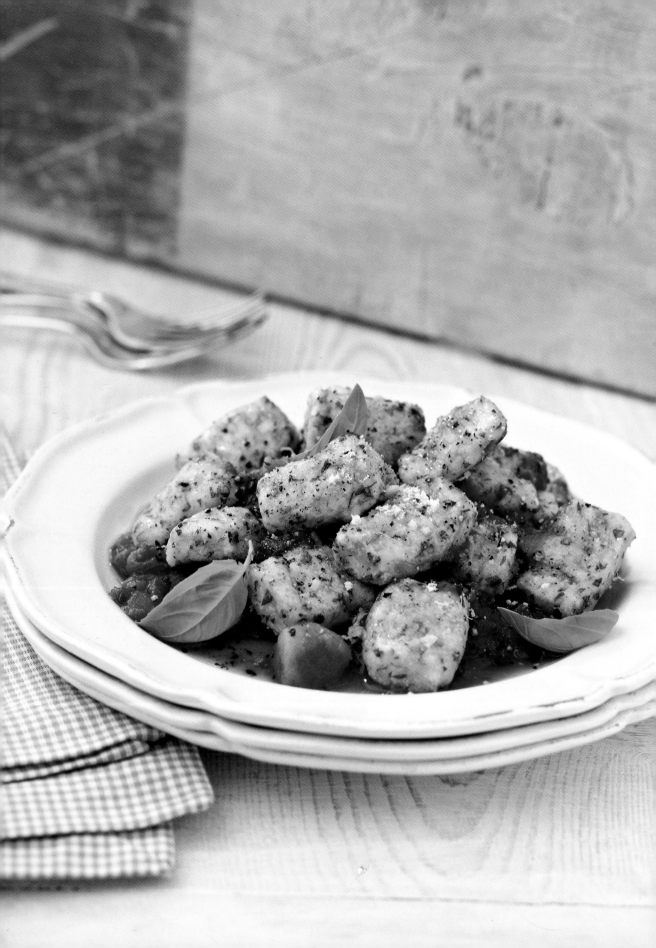

Baked gnocchi

These light and fluffy potato dumplings are flavoured with parsley and accompanied with an Italian-style basil-flavoured sauce.

SERVES 4

EASY (V) (✱)

Syns per serving
Extra Easy: 3½
Green: 3½
Original: 11

Preparation time 25 minutes plus overnight chilling
Cooking time under 30 minutes

800g/1lb 12oz boiled potatoes
8 tbsp finely chopped parsley
¼ tsp freshly grated nutmeg
1 small egg, beaten
salt and freshly ground black pepper
2 x 400g cans chopped tomatoes
1 onion, peeled and finely diced
3 garlic cloves, peeled and crushed
4 tbsp finely chopped basil
100g/3½oz reduced fat Cheddar cheese, grated
a few basil leaves
Parmesan cheese, grated (optional)

TO SERVE
a crisp green salad (optional)

Place the potatoes in a bowl with the parsley, nutmeg and egg. Season well and mash thoroughly until well combined. Cover and chill in the fridge overnight.

Preheat the oven to 190°C/Gas 5. Place the tomatoes, onion, garlic and basil in a saucepan and bring to the boil. Cook over a high heat for 10–12 minutes, stirring occasionally, season well and remove from the heat. Spoon this mixture over the base of a medium-sized, shallow ovenproof dish.

Make the gnocchi by making small, walnut-sized balls from the potato mixture and place them in a single layer over the tomatoes. Sprinkle over the grated cheese and bake in the oven for 10 minutes until hot and bubbling. Garnish with the basil leaves, sprinkle with Parmesan (1½ Syns per tablespoon), if using, and serve immediately with a crisp green salad, if wished.

Pasta al funghi

SERVES 4

EASY

Syns per serving
Extra Easy: ½
Green: 2
Original: 10

Preparation time 5 minutes
plus soaking
Cooking time 10–12 minutes

225g/8oz dried pasta shapes or tubes
low calorie cooking spray
450g/1lb mushrooms, sliced
75g/3oz lean bacon, cut into cubes
a pinch of freshly grated nutmeg
150g/5oz fat free natural fromage frais
salt and freshly ground black pepper
2 tbsp finely chopped flat-leaf parsley
1 tbsp grated Parmesan cheese

TO SERVE
a mixed salad

You can use any fresh mushrooms in this recipe but wild or chestnut ones have a more intense flavour than button mushrooms.

Cook the pasta according to the packet instructions until just tender. Drain well.

While the pasta is cooking, spray a large non-stick frying pan with low calorie cooking spray and place it over a low heat. When the pan is hot, add the mushrooms and bacon and cook for about 5 minutes, until golden brown. Over a very low heat, stir in the nutmeg, gently fold in the fromage frais, heat through and season to taste.

Tip the drained pasta into the pan and toss gently to coat evenly with the sauce. Sprinkle with the parsley and Parmesan, and serve immediately with a mixed salad.

Tagliatelle Napoletana

SERVES 4

EASY (V)

Syns per serving
Extra Easy: 1/2
Green: 1/2
Original: 10½

Preparation time 10 minutes
Cooking time 30 minutes

450g/1lb tomatoes
low calorie cooking spray
1 large onion, peeled and chopped
2 garlic cloves, peeled and crushed
1 tbsp chopped oregano
16 black olives
1 tbsp of capers, drained
225g/8oz dried tagliatelle
2 tbsp chopped basil or flat-leaf
parsley

In this recipe, the ribbons of tender pasta are topped with a roasted tomato sauce fragrant with Mediterranean herbs and salty black olives.

Preheat the oven to 180°C/Gas 4. Put the tomatoes in a roasting tin and bake for 12–15 minutes, until softened and the skins are slightly charred. Remove the skins and roughly chop the flesh.

Spray a large non-stick saucepan with low calorie cooking spray and place over a medium heat. Add the onion and garlic and sauté gently for about 5 minutes, until soft and golden. Add the tomatoes, oregano, olives and capers, and simmer gently for about 10 minutes, until slightly thickened.

Meanwhile, cook the tagliatelle according to the packet instructions until just tender. Drain thoroughly and divide between four serving plates. Top with the tomato sauce and sprinkle with the basil or parsley. Serve immediately.

Italian grilled squid with gremolata

Gremolata is a mixture of finely chopped parsley, lemon zest and garlic, and is used as a final seasoning for many fish and meat dishes. Here it is tossed with grilled squid for a very tasty supper.

SERVES 4

EASY

Syns per serving
Extra Easy: Free
Original: Free
Green: 5

Preparation time 25 minutes
Cooking time 5–6 minutes

8 medium squid, with tentacles, cleaned
salt and freshly ground black pepper

FOR THE GREMOLATA
25g/1oz flat-leaf parsley, chopped
25g/1oz mint, chopped
1 red chilli, deseeded and finely chopped
4 garlic cloves, peeled and finely chopped
4 tbsp small capers, drained
2 tbsp finely grated lemon zest

TO SERVE
50g/2oz rocket leaves
lemon wedges

Preheat the grill to hot.

Cut the squid open and flatten the pieces. Using a sharp knife, score diamond patterns on the inner side of the squid body. Season the squid and tentacles and place, scored sides down, under the grill. Cook for 1–2 minutes.

Turn the squid pieces over – they'll start to curl up almost straight away, by which time they will be cooked. Remove from the grill and place in a bowl.

To make the gremolata, place the herbs, chilli, garlic, capers and lemon zest in a bowl and mix to combine. Season well and spoon over the grilled squid. Toss to mix well.

Divide the rocket leaves between four plates and top with the squid. Serve with lemon wedges to squeeze over.

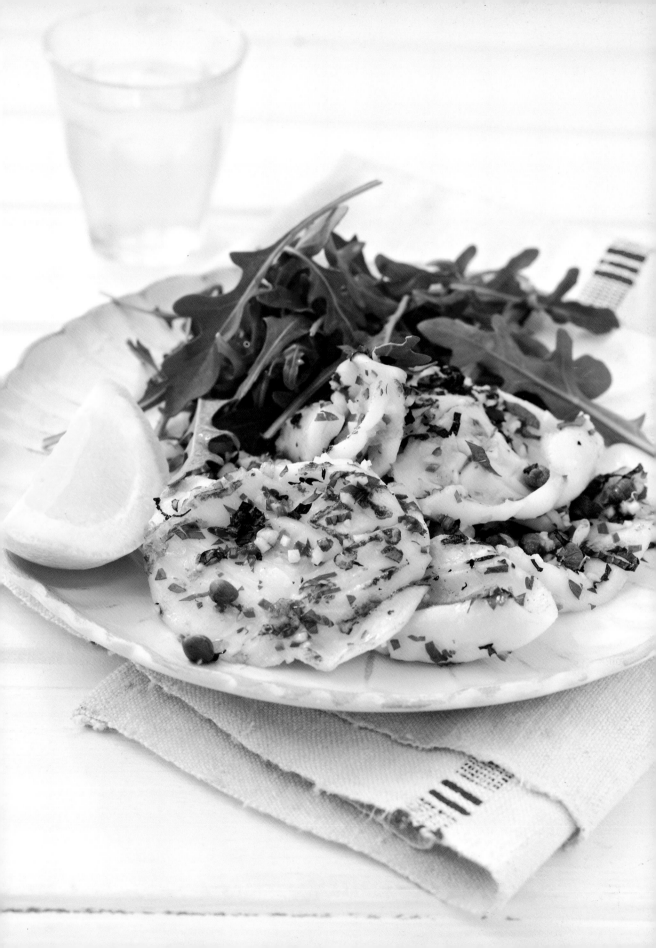

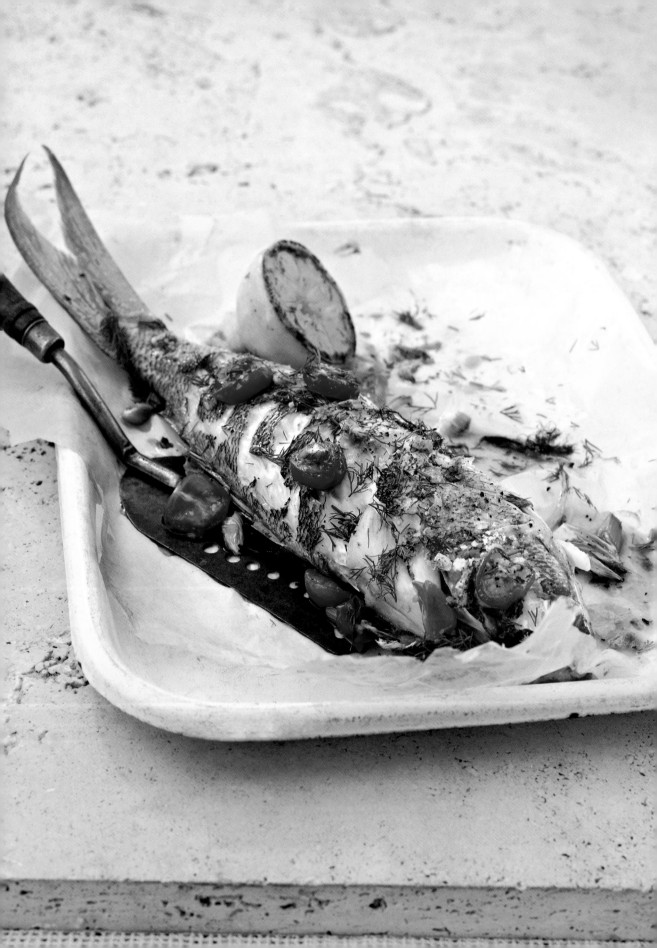

Red mullet al cartoccio

SERVES 4

EASY ❄ (only if fish are fresh)

Syns per serving
Extra Easy: Free
Original: Free
Green: 20

Preparation time 15–20 minutes
Cooking time 15–20 minutes

1 large fennel bulb, trimmed
and finely sliced
10 cherry tomatoes,
halved or quartered
4 tbsp lemon juice
2 garlic cloves, peeled and sliced
4 x 350g/12oz red mullet,
cleaned and scaled
salt and freshly ground black pepper

TO SERVE
chopped dill or fennel fronds

'Al cartoccio' is the Italian term for 'cooking in a bag' where ingredients are sealed in a foil or baking parchment parcel and cooked, steaming in their own juices and flavours.

Preheat the oven to 220°C/Gas 7. Cut four pieces of foil or baking parchment, each four times the length of the red mullet.

In a bowl, mix the fennel with the tomatoes, lemon juice and garlic. Divide half the fennel mixture equally between the centre of each piece of foil or parchment.

Cut the skin of the red mullet three or four times on each side and season both sides well. Place the fish on top of the fennel mixture.

Spoon the remaining fennel mixture over the fish portions and bring together the edges of the foil or parchment to form loose parcels. Seal the edges by folding tightly and place the parcels on two large baking sheets.

Bake in the oven for 15–20 minutes. Transfer the parcels to serving plates and leave to stand for 5 minutes. Split the parcels open, garnish with chopped dill or fennel fronds and serve immediately.

Ham and egg linguine

SERVES 4

EASY

Syns per serving
Extra Easy: ½
Green: 2½
Original: 10

Preparation time 5 minutes
Cooking time 8–14 minutes

225g/8oz dried linguine or spaghetti
low calorie cooking spray
4 eggs
1 tbsp grated Parmesan cheese
2 tbsp chopped flat-leaf parsley
salt and freshly ground black pepper
110g/4oz cooked ham, diced

This recipe is a variation on the Italian spaghetti carbonara. The linguine are tossed with a little grated Parmesan cheese and some parsley, then scattered with diced ham and topped with a fried egg. Delicious!

Cook the pasta according to the packet instructions until tender but still a little firm. Stir occasionally while it is cooking to prevent the strands of pasta sticking together. Drain well and return to the pan.

Meanwhile, spray a non-stick frying pan with low calorie cooking spray and fry the eggs in batches until the whites are set but the yolks are still runny. Remove from the pan and keep warm.

Toss the cooked pasta with the Parmesan and parsley. Season, stir in the ham and divide between four plates. Top each serving with a fried egg and serve immediately.

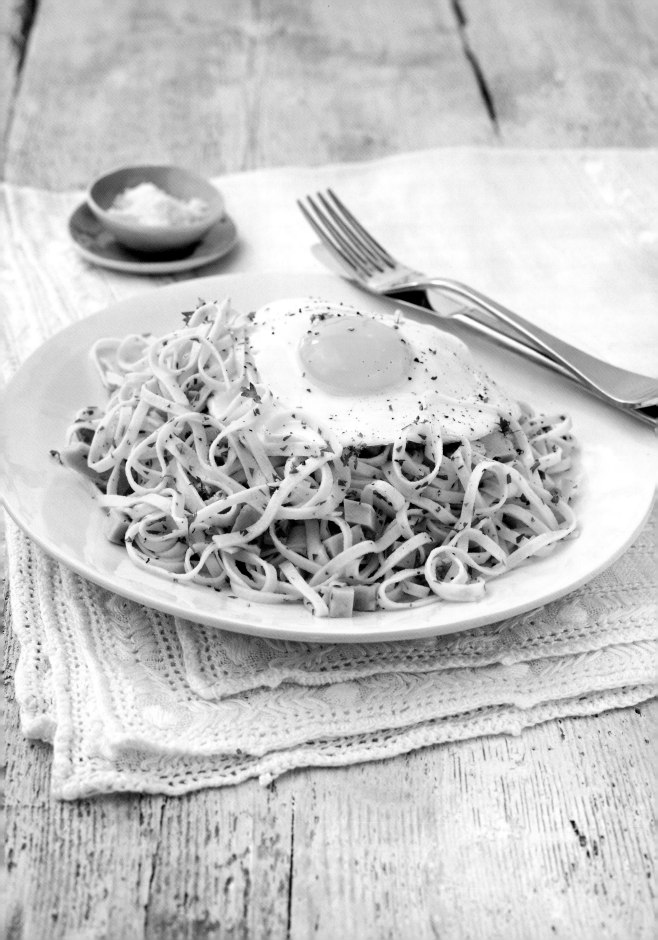

Italian meatballs in tomato sauce

For a really authentic Italian meal, you can serve these little meatballs on a bed of spaghetti.

SERVES 4

EASY ❄

Syns per serving
Extra Easy: Free
Original: Free
Green: 7½

Preparation time 15 minutes
Cooking time 25 minutes

350g/12oz extra lean minced beef
½ small onion, peeled and grated
2 garlic cloves, peeled and crushed
½ tsp ground cumin
2 tbsp chopped flat-leaf parsley
salt and freshly ground black pepper
1 egg, beaten

FOR THE TOMATO SAUCE
1 onion, peeled and finely chopped
2 garlic cloves, peeled and crushed
400g can chopped tomatoes
1 tbsp tomato purée
1 tsp chopped basil or oregano
salt and freshly ground black pepper
½ tsp artificial sweetener

TO SERVE
chopped flat-leaf parsley
a crisp salad

To make the meatballs, put the minced beef, onion, garlic, cumin, parsley and seasoning in a large bowl and mix together well. Bind with the beaten egg, divide into 16 portions and roll each one into a ball.

Preheat the grill to hot. Place the meatballs under the grill and cook for about 10 minutes, until they are starting to brown.

Meanwhile, make the tomato sauce. Put all the ingredients in a large saucepan, cover and bring to the boil. Reduce the heat and allow to simmer gently for 10 minutes.

Add the meatballs to the tomato sauce in the pan, cover and cook gently over a low heat for about 15 minutes, until the meat is thoroughly cooked. Serve sprinkled with the parsley and accompany with a crisp salad.

Tuscan chicken

SERVES 4

EASY ❄

Syns per serving
Extra Easy: 1½
Original: 1½
Green: 6

Preparation time 10 minutes
Cooking time 50–60 minutes

1 onion, peeled and chopped
175g/6oz button mushrooms
2 garlic cloves, peeled and crushed
300ml/½ pint chicken stock
225g/8oz plum tomatoes, skinned and
chopped
a few rosemary sprigs
150ml/¼ pint red wine
8 skinless chicken thighs
salt and freshly ground black pepper

TO SERVE
2 tbsp chopped flat-leaf parsley
vegetables of your choice

Tuscan cooking is simple and doesn't use the heavy sauces found in other regions. This variation on a traditional recipe is warming on a winter's day.

Put the onion, mushrooms, garlic and stock in a heavy-based saucepan, cover and bring to the boil. Continue boiling for 5–10 minutes, then uncover, lower the heat and simmer gently for 20–30 minutes until the vegetables are golden and cooked, and the liquid has been absorbed.

Add the tomatoes, rosemary and red wine, stirring well, and then add the chicken and season to taste. Cover the pan and simmer gently for about 20 minutes until the chicken is thoroughly cooked. Check the pan from time to time to ensure the sauce does not stick and get too dry. Add more stock if necessary.

Serve the Tuscan chicken sprinkled with the parsley and accompanied with vegetables of your choice.

Veal saltimbocca

SERVES 4

EASY ✳

Syns per serving
Extra Easy: 2
Original: 2
Green: 14½

Preparation time 20 minutes
Cooking time about 20 minutes

4 x 200g lean veal escalopes
freshly ground black pepper
8 sage leaves
4 very thin slices of Parma ham
low calorie cooking spray
3 tbsp Marsala or any Italian red wine
240ml/8fl oz chicken stock
1 tbsp gravy granules

TO SERVE
lemon wedges (optional)
green beans

For this classic Italian dish, the veal escalopes are pounded to be as thin as possible then wrapped in Parma ham and cooked in a red wine sauce. Thin pork escalopes can successfully replace the veal in this recipe if desired.

Place the veal escalopes between sheets of cling film and, using a mallet or rolling pin, beat lightly until about 1cm/½in thick. Remove the cling film and season the veal very well with freshly ground black pepper.

Lay out the escalopes on a clean work surface. Place two sage leaves on each escalope and wrap each one with a slice of Parma ham.

Spray a large non-stick frying pan with low calorie cooking spray and place over a high heat. Add the escalopes and cook on each side for 3–4 minutes or until just cooked through. Using a slotted spoon, remove from the pan and keep warm.

Add the Marsala or red wine to the pan and cook over a high heat for 30–40 seconds, then add the stock and granules, bring to the boil and cook for 4–5 minutes. Reduce the heat, return the veal to the pan, spoon over the Marsala mixture and heat through.

To serve, place each escalope in the centre of a warmed plate and spoon over the reduced stock mixture. Garnish with lemon wedges, if using, and serve, accompanied with green beans.

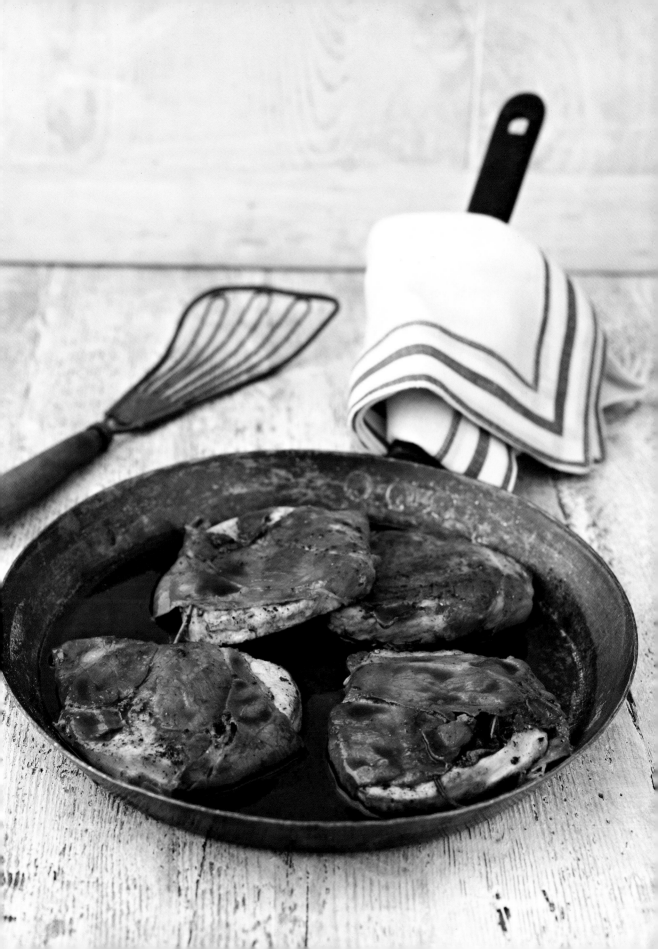

Tiramisù pots

SERVES 4

EASY (V) (❄)

Syns per serving
Extra Easy: 2
Original: 2
Green: 2

Preparation time 15 minutes plus chilling

4 sponge fingers
200ml/7fl oz cooled espresso coffee
200g/7oz quark
200g/7oz fat free natural fromage frais plus 4 tbsp for the topping
4–5 tbsp artificial sweetener
1 tsp vanilla extract
200g/7oz fat free vanilla yogurt
4 tbsp low fat custard
1 tsp cocoa powder, to dust

First made popular in the 1980s, this 'pud' has never gone out of fashion. Leave the desserts in the fridge while the biscuits soak up the espresso, or serve them immediately for a crunchier finish.

Chop the sponge fingers into smallish pieces (do not break them up too much as you want to retain some crunch) and place in a bowl. Pour the espresso over the top. Once the coffee has been absorbed, divide half the mixture between four dessert glasses.

In another bowl, mix together the quark, fromage frais, sweetener, vanilla extract and yogurt until smooth. Spoon half this mixture over the biscuit mixtures in the glasses.

Repeat the layering with the remaining biscuit mixture and quark mixture, finishing with one tablespoonful of custard in each glass. Place the glasses in the fridge for 2–3 hours if you want the sponge fingers to soak up the espresso, or until chilled.

Spoon one tablespoon of fromage frais over each dessert, dust with the cocoa powder and serve.

Zabaglione

SERVES 4

WORTH THE EFFORT (V)

Syns per serving
Extra Easy: 6
Original: 6
Green: 6

Preparation time 2 minutes
Cooking time 10–15 minutes

4 egg yolks
5 tbsp caster sugar
120ml/4fl oz Marsala

To achieve the best and most authentic result with this sensational dessert, you must use real Marsala, a fortified wine that is available in most supermarkets. Zabaglione can be served hot, in the traditional way, or chilled.

Put the egg yolks in the top of a double boiler, or in a basin standing over a small saucepan of gently simmering water. The basin should not be in direct contact with the water below.

Stir the sugar and Marsala into the egg yolks, and then start beating with a wire whisk or an electric hand-held whisk, until the mixture is thick and hot. Be patient – this process cannot be rushed, and it may take about 10 minutes, but the end result will make it all worthwhile. While you are whisking, the water should continue to simmer – make sure that it does not boil dry.

Spoon the hot zabaglione into four tall glasses and serve immediately.

Alternatively, you can allow the mixture to cool completely, then put some sliced strawberries or peaches in four serving dishes and spoon the cold zabaglione on top.

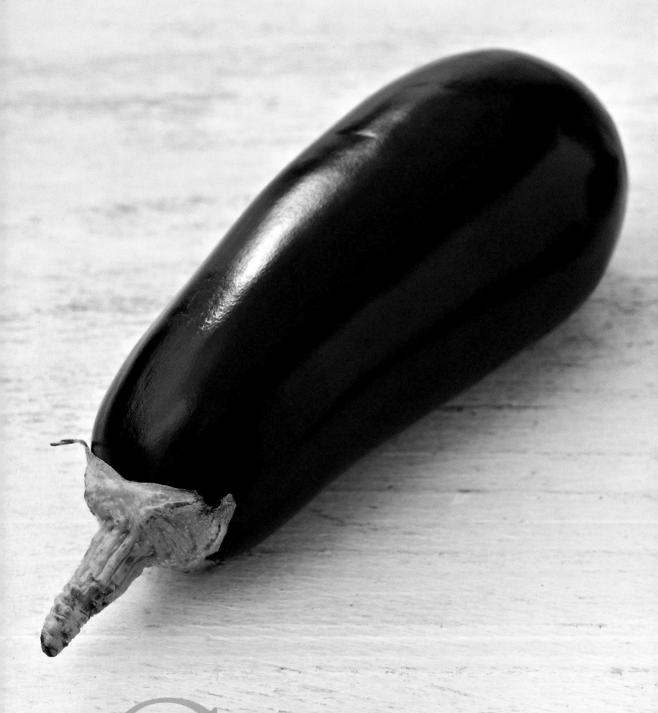

Greece

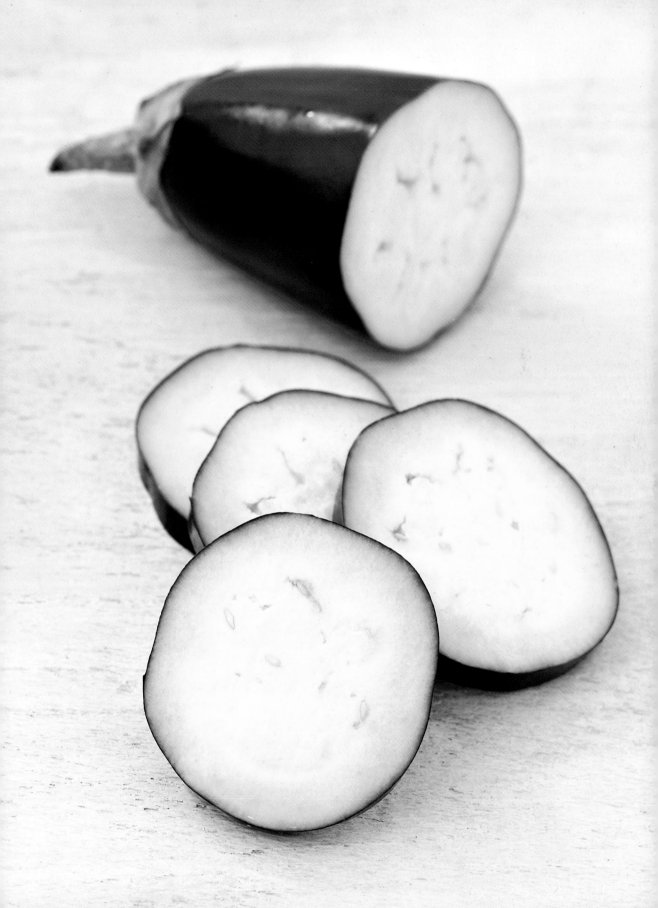

Trio of Greek dips

These wonderful dips can be prepared in advance and make for a lovely starter to any picnic or casual summer's lunch. Serve them with vegetable crudités cut from carrots, celery sticks and cucumber.

SERVES 4

EASY Ⓥ ❄

Syns per serving
Extra Easy: Free
Original: Free
Green: Free

Preparation time 10 minutes
Cooking time 15 minutes

2 large aubergines
2 garlic cloves, peeled
1 tsp salt
1 small handful thyme
2 tbsp lemon juice
2 heaped tbsp low fat natural Greek yogurt
salt and freshly ground black pepper

TO SERVE
a pinch of paprika
chopped flat-leaf parsley

AUBERGINE DIP
Preheat the grill to high. Prick the aubergines with a fork and grill them, turning occasionally, until the skin blisters and blackens all over. Remove from the grill and, when cool, peel off the skin. Leave the aubergine flesh in a colander for 15 minutes to drain off excess liquid.

Pound the garlic and salt until smooth with a pestle and mortar. Transfer to a food processor. Add the aubergine flesh, thyme, lemon juice and yogurt. Whizz to a thick purée and adjust the seasoning. Transfer to a bowl, sprinkle with the paprika and chopped parsley and serve.

(continues over)

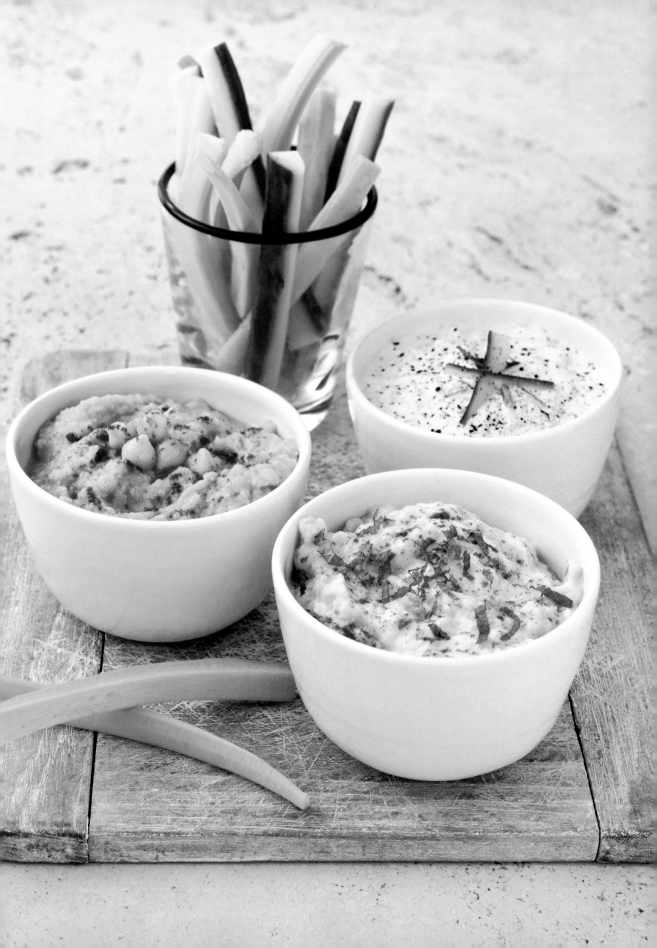

SERVES 4

EASY (V) (❄)

Syns per serving
Extra Easy: ½
Original: ½
Green: ½

Preparation time 10 minutes

1 cucumber, peeled, deseeded
and coarsely grated
200g/7oz low fat natural Greek yogurt
4 garlic cloves, peeled and crushed
a small handful of mint, chopped
1 tbsp lemon juice
salt and freshly ground black pepper

TZATZIKI

Mix the cucumber with the yogurt, garlic, mint and lemon juice and season well. Transfer to a serving bowl and chill until ready to serve.

SERVES 4

EASY (V) (❄)

Syns per serving
Extra Easy: Free
Green: Free
Original: 3

Preparation time 10 minutes

200g/7oz canned chickpeas, drained
and rinsed
juice of ½ lemon
2 garlic cloves, peeled and crushed
2 tsp ground cumin
salt and freshly ground black pepper
1 tsp sweet smoked paprika

HOUMOUS

Combine the chickpeas, lemon juice, garlic, cumin and 120ml/4fl oz of water in a food processor, and blitz until smooth and creamy. Season well.

Turn out into a serving bowl, and sprinkle with paprika before serving.

Mushrooms à la grecque

SERVES 4

EASY Ⓥ

Syns per serving
Extra Easy: ½
Original: ½
Green: ½

Preparation time 10 minutes
Cooking time 10 minutes

low calorie cooking spray
2 large onions, peeled and sliced
2 garlic cloves, peeled
and finely chopped
600g/1lb 6oz button
mushrooms, halved
8 plum tomatoes, roughly chopped
16 black olives, sliced
2 garlic cloves, peeled and crushed
2 tbsp white wine vinegar
salt and freshly ground black pepper

This delicious mushroom salad can be made up to a day in advance and chilled in the fridge. Just make sure it comes back to room temperature before serving.

Spray a large non-stick frying pan with low calorie cooking spray and place over a medium heat. Fry the onions and chopped garlic until soft and starting to brown. Add the mushrooms and tomatoes and gently stir-fry for 4–5 minutes. Remove from the heat. Place in a serving dish and scatter over the olives.

Mix the crushed garlic with the vinegar, season and drizzle over the mushrooms. Cover and allow to stand for 30 minutes at room temperature before serving.

Dolmades

SERVES 6

WORTH THE EFFORT Ⓥ ❋

Syns per serving
Extra Easy: ½
Green: ½
Original: 4

Preparation time 15 minutes plus
soaking
Cooking time 1½ hours

175g/6oz pickled vine leaves
110g/4oz dried long-grain rice
1 small onion, peeled
and finely chopped
1 tomato, skinned, deseeded
and chopped
a few parsley sprigs, chopped
1 tbsp chopped mint
a pinch each of ground cinnamon,
allspice and cumin
salt and freshly ground black pepper
3 garlic cloves, peeled and sliced
juice of 2 lemons
1 tsp olive oil

TO SERVE
lemon wedges (optional)
pickled chillies (optional)

These lemon-scented appetisers are served throughout Greece as a snack, or mezze. You can buy pickled vine leaves in packets or jars in most supermarkets and delicatessens.

Soak the vine leaves in hot water for 20–30 minutes. Remove, drain and pat dry with kitchen paper. Remove the stalks from the leaves and spread out the leaves on a clean work surface, with the veined sides facing upwards.

Soak the rice in boiling water for a few minutes, then drain. In a bowl, mix the rice with the onion, tomato, herbs and spices, and season.

Place a little of this mixture in the centre of each vine leaf, then fold the sides of the leaf over into the middle to encase the filling, and roll up like a cigar.

Line the base of a large saucepan with any broken or leftover leaves and pack the dolmades in tightly, in layers. Tuck in the garlic slices among them, cover with 150ml/¼ pint of water and the lemon juice and oil, and press a heatproof plate down on top.

Cover the saucepan and simmer gently for 1½ hours, checking occasionally that there is still enough liquid to cover the dolmades and adding more water if necessary.

Leave the dolmades in the pan to cool, then remove and serve cold. Accompany with lemon wedges and pickled chillies, if wished.

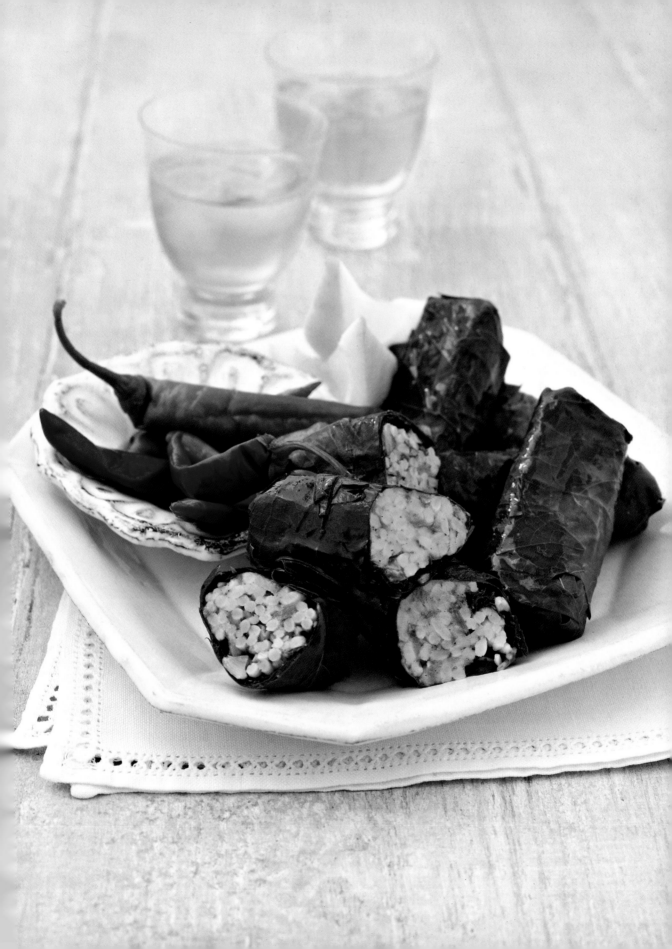

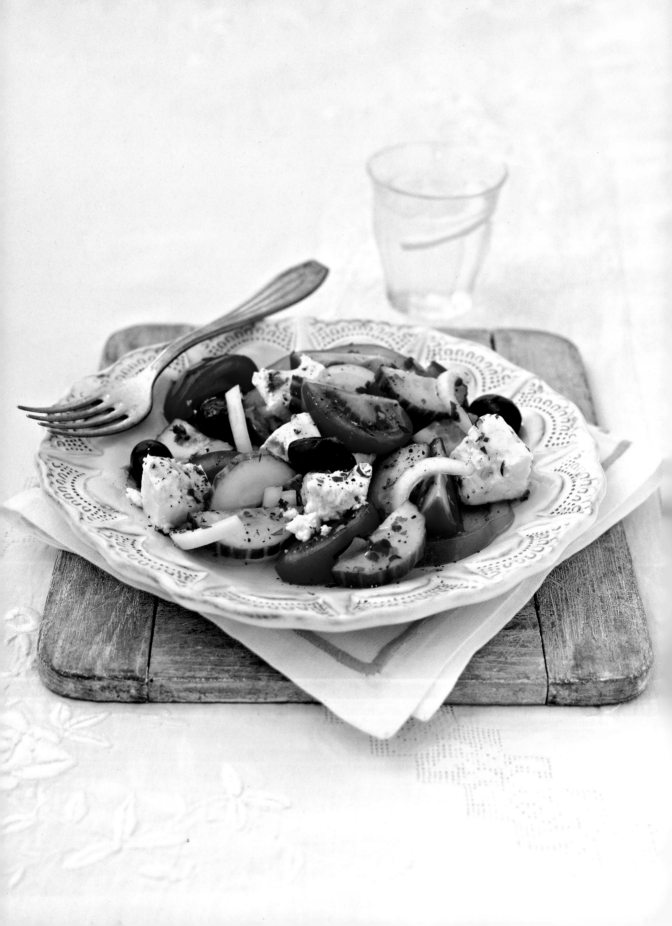

Greek-style feta salad

SERVES 4

EXTRA EASY Ⓥ

Syns per serving
Extra Easy: 3½
Original: 3½
Green: 3½

Preparation time 15 minutes

4 tomatoes, cut into wedges
½ cucumber, halved lengthways
and sliced
1 green pepper, deseeded and cut
into rings or thinly sliced
1 onion, peeled and cut into
thinly sliced rings
110g/4oz reduced fat feta cheese,
cut into cubes
8 black olives
salt and freshly ground black pepper
4 tbsp fat free salad dressing
a bunch of flat-leaf parsley, chopped

This refreshing, crisp salad evokes all the flavours, colours and textures of the Mediterranean. Try adding watermelon cubes to it for a typical Greek-style variation.

Arrange the tomatoes, cucumber, green pepper and onion in a serving dish. Top with the feta and olives.

Season well and drizzle the dressing over the top. Sprinkle with the parsley and serve immediately.

Grilled halloumi and vegetable skewers

SERVES 4

EASY Ⓥ

Syns per serving
Extra Easy: 4½
Original: 4½
Green: 4½

Preparation time 10 minutes
Cooking time about 8 minutes

2 red peppers, deseeded and
cut into bite-sized pieces
1 yellow pepper, deseeded and
cut into bite-sized pieces
2 medium red onions, peeled
and cut into wedges
110g/4oz firm halloumi cheese,
cut into bite-sized pieces
low calorie cooking spray
salt and freshly ground black pepper
2 tsp dried mixed herbs

TO SERVE
finely chopped flat-leaf parsley

Due to its high melting point, flavoursome halloumi cheese is perfect for grilling under a hot grill or on the barbecue.

Thread the peppers, onions and halloumi evenly and alternately between eight medium-sized metal skewers. Spray with low calorie cooking spray and season well.

Preheat the grill to medium–hot, or prepare the barbecue. Sprinkle the mixed herbs over the skewers and place them on a grill rack under the grill or on the barbecue. Cook for 3–4 minutes on each side or until lightly browned at the edges. Remove from the heat and sprinkle with the parsley before serving.

Greek vegetable casserole

SERVES 4

EASY (V) (❄)

Syns per serving
Extra Easy: 5
Original: 5
Green: 5

Preparation time 10 minutes
Cooking time 20 minutes

low calorie cooking spray
1 onion, peeled and cut into thinly
sliced rings
3 peppers of mixed colours, deseeded
and cut into rings
4 garlic cloves, peeled and crushed
4 tomatoes, chopped
200g/7oz reduced fat feta cheese, cut
into cubes
1 tsp oregano
salt and freshly ground black pepper

The flavours of Greece come alive in this simple and tasty dish of peppers, tomatoes and vegetables, flavoured with aromatic oregano and creamy feta cheese.

Preheat the oven to 200°C/Gas 6. Spray a large non-stick frying pan with low calorie cooking spray and place over a medium heat. Stir-fry the onion, peppers and garlic until soft and starting to brown.

Add the tomatoes and cook for a few more minutes to soften. Transfer to an ovenproof dish and mix in the feta and oregano. Season, cover tightly and bake in the oven for 15 minutes. Serve immediately.

Greek souvlakia

SERVES 4

EASY ❄

Syns per serving
Extra Easy: Free
Original: Free
Green: 6½

Preparation time 10 minutes
plus marinating
Cooking time 4–5 minutes

1 onion, peeled and grated
2 garlic cloves, peeled and crushed
2 tbsp each chopped oregano
and rosemary
1 tsp ground cumin
1 tsp cayenne pepper
juice of 1 lemon
salt and freshly ground black pepper
350g/12oz lean lamb fillet,
cut into small cubes

FOR THE MINTY YOGURT
150g/5oz fat free natural yogurt
2 spring onions, trimmed
and thinly sliced
1 tbsp chopped mint
a few coriander leaves, chopped
salt and freshly ground black pepper

TO SERVE
a crisp mixed salad

Tender lamb grilled with fragrant Mediterranean herbs and garlic is a popular feature of Greek cookery. Crisp lettuce, spring onions, sliced juicy tomatoes and chunks of cucumber go really well with this dish.

In a large bowl, mix together the onion, garlic, herbs, cumin, cayenne pepper, lemon juice and seasoning. Add the lamb and stir gently until it is completely coated in the marinade mixture. Set aside in a cool place for about 1 hour.

Preheat the grill to hot. Remove the lamb from the marinade, transfer to a baking sheet and cook under the grill for 4–5 minutes, until crisp and a little charred. Turn the lamb cubes over occasionally so that they cook evenly. Do not overcook; ideally, the lamb should still be pink and juicy inside.

While the lamb is cooking, mix together the minty yogurt ingredients in a bowl. Serve the souvlakia with the yogurt and a crisp salad.

Stifado

SERVES 4

EASY ✳

Syns per serving
Extra Easy: 1½
Original: 1½
Green: 9

Preparation time 15 minutes
Cooking time 2½–3 hours

2 onions, peeled and sliced
3 garlic cloves, peeled and crushed
600ml/1 pint beef stock
450g/1lb lean stewing steak,
cut into cubes
1 tbsp tomato purée
180ml/6fl oz red wine
2 tbsp red wine vinegar
2 thyme sprigs
1 rosemary sprig
1 bay leaf
½ tsp cumin seeds
½ tsp cloves
1 cinnamon stick
450g/1lb pickling onions,
peeled and blanched
juice of ½ lemon
salt and freshly ground black pepper

TO SERVE
2 tbsp chopped coriander

Stifado is an aromatic stew of beef and vegetables cooked in red wine with herbs and is a popular Greek dish. Don't forget the red wine vinegar, which is a vital ingredient in flavouring the stifado.

Put the onions, garlic and half of the stock in a large flameproof casserole dish. Cover and bring to the boil for 5–10 minutes, then reduce the heat and simmer uncovered for 20–30 minutes, until the onions are tender and golden.

Add the steak and cook over a low heat, turning occasionally, until browned all over. Stir in the tomato purée, red wine, vinegar and herbs and the remaining stock.

Preheat the oven to 170°C/Gas 3. Tie the cumin seeds, cloves and cinnamon stick in a piece of muslin and place in the dish. Cover and cook in the oven for 2–2½ hours until the steak is tender, adding the pickling onions after 1 hour.

Remove the herbs and spice bag from the casserole. Add the lemon juice and seasoning, sprinkle with the coriander and serve.

Lamb moussaka

2 large aubergines, thinly sliced
salt
low calorie cooking spray
2 onions, peeled and chopped
500g/1lb 2oz extra lean minced lamb
400g can chopped tomatoes
1 tbsp chopped oregano
(or 1 tsp dried)
½ tsp each of ground cinnamon,
allspice and cumin
2 tbsp tomato purée
60ml/2fl oz red wine
salt and freshly ground black pepper

FOR THE TOPPING
150g/5oz fat free natural yogurt
2 eggs, beaten
60ml/2fl oz skimmed milk

TO SERVE
a crisp salad

Moussaka is usually high in Syns, but this low-Syn version tastes wonderful and lacks the oiliness of the traditionally made dish.

Put the aubergines in a colander and sprinkle generously with salt. Leave for at least 30 minutes to drain away their bitter moisture. Rinse and pat dry with kitchen paper.

Spray a large non-stick frying pan with low calorie cooking spray and place over a medium heat. Fry the aubergine slices in batches until slightly coloured, then remove and set aside.

Spray the pan with low calorie cooking spray and add the onions and lamb. Cook gently until the mince is browned. Add the tomatoes, oregano, spices and tomato purée. Bring to the boil and cook rapidly until the sauce thickens. Stir in the red wine and bring back to the boil. Season well.

Arrange a third of the aubergine slices in a shallow ovenproof dish. Cover with half the meat sauce and repeat the layers, finishing with aubergine slices.

Preheat the oven to 180°C/Gas 4. Beat together the topping ingredients, season and pour over the moussaka. Bake in the oven for about 30 minutes, until the topping is set, golden and slightly risen. Serve immediately with a crisp salad.

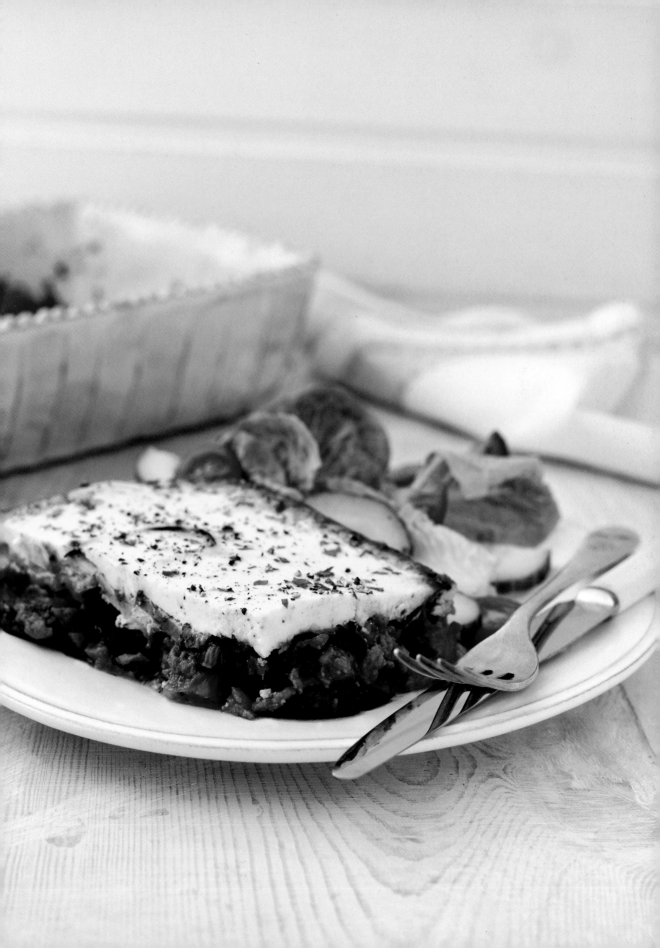

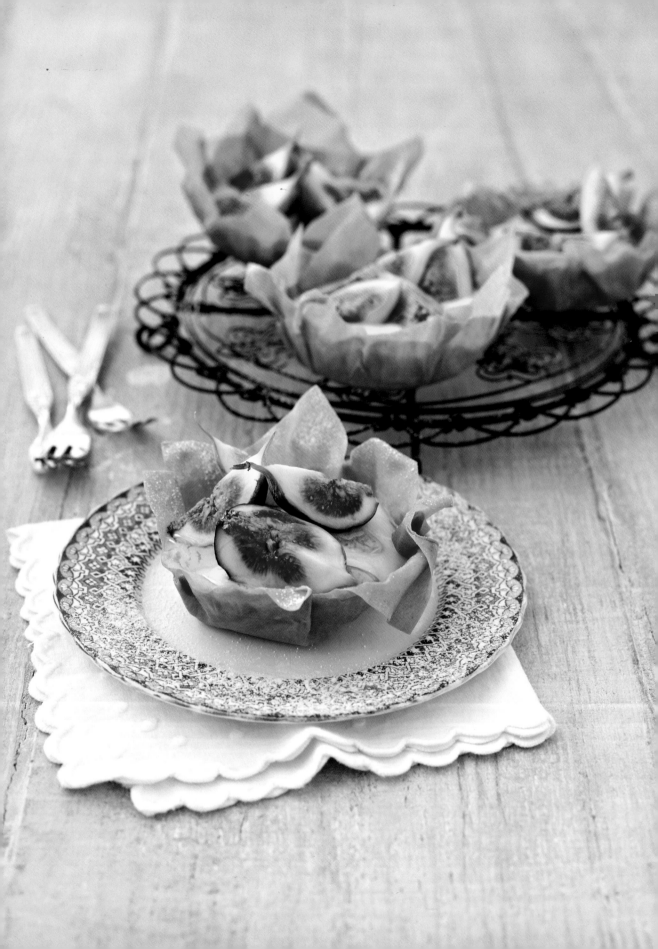

Greek filo and fig cups

SERVES 4

WORTH THE EFFORT Ⓥ

Syns per serving
Extra Easy: 3
Original: 3
Green: 3

Preparation time 15 minutes
Cooking time 8–10 minutes

1 large sheet filo pastry, approx 45 x
25cm (18 x 10in)
low calorie cooking spray
4 tbsp low fat custard
4 ripe figs
4 tsp clear honey
1 tsp icing sugar

Fresh figs, custard, crisp filo pastry and a little drizzle of honey make this dessert so very moreish.

Preheat the oven to 200°C/Gas 6. Cut the filo sheet in half and cut each half into four squares so that you have eight 12cm/4½in squares. Spray each square with a little low calorie cooking spray and use a pastry brush to spread it evenly over the squares.

Spray the insides of four non-stick individual tartlet tins with low calorie cooking spray and use the pastry brush to spread the spray evenly.

Line each tin with two filo squares stacked at a 90° angle. Bake the filo cups for 8–10 minutes, until crispy and golden. Allow to cool, then remove from the tins.

To serve, place one tablespoon of the custard in each filo cup. Cut each fig into quarters, place on top of the custard and drizzle with one teaspoon of honey. Lightly dust with the icing sugar and serve immediately.

Lemon and honey granita

Granita originally came from Sicily and is a semi-frozen dessert of sugar, water and flavourings, not unlike a sorbet. It is perfect for a hot summer's day.

SERVES 8 (makes about 500ml/18fl oz)

EASY (V) (❄)

Syns per serving
Extra Easy: ½
Original: ½
Green: ½

Preparation time 15 minutes plus freezing

6–8 tbsp artificial sweetener
4 lemons
2 tbsp clear honey

Put the sweetener and 400ml/14fl oz of water into a saucepan. Using a zester or vegetable peeler, thinly pare strips of the zest from one of the lemons and add to the pan.

Heat gently, stirring until the sweetener has completely dissolved. Bring to the boil and then remove from the heat and leave to cool. When cold, strain into a large shallow plastic container. Juice all the lemons and stir into the syrup along with the honey.

Freeze for 2 hours. Remove from the freezer and mash up any crystals that have formed with a fork. Return to the freezer for another 2 hours and repeat the mashing. Freeze for at least 1 more hour before serving.

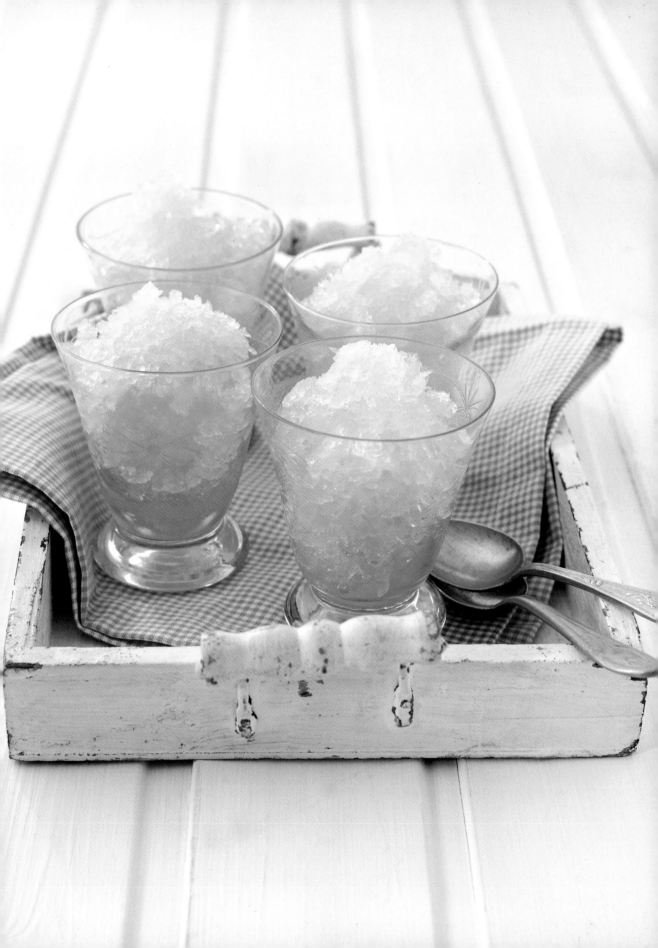

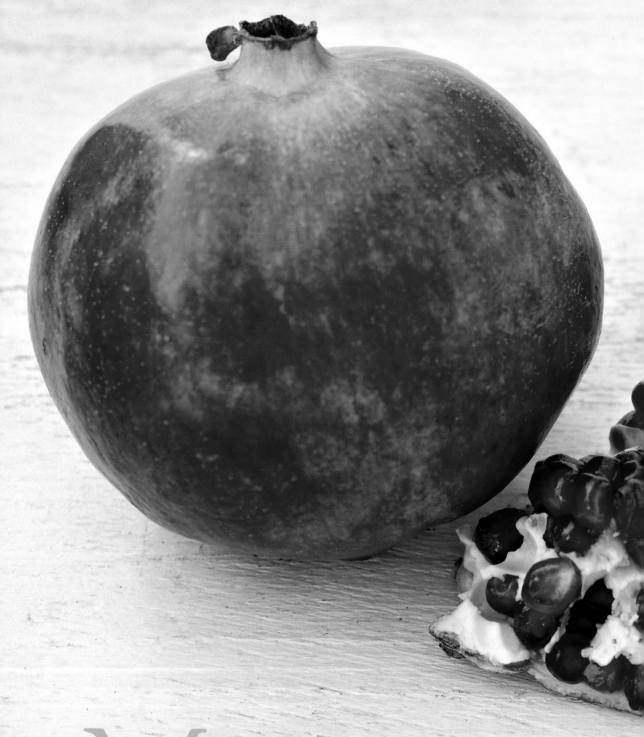

Morocco

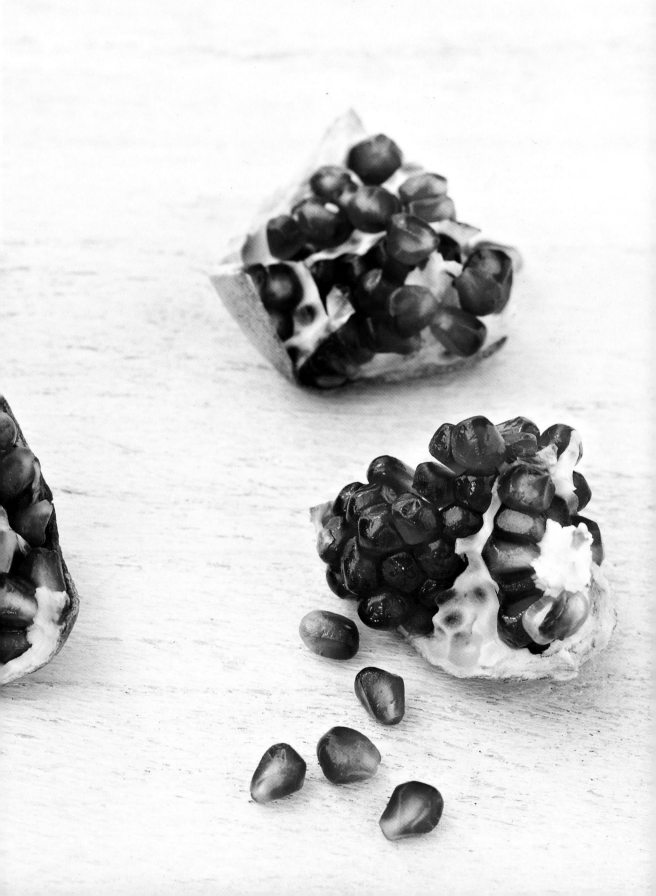

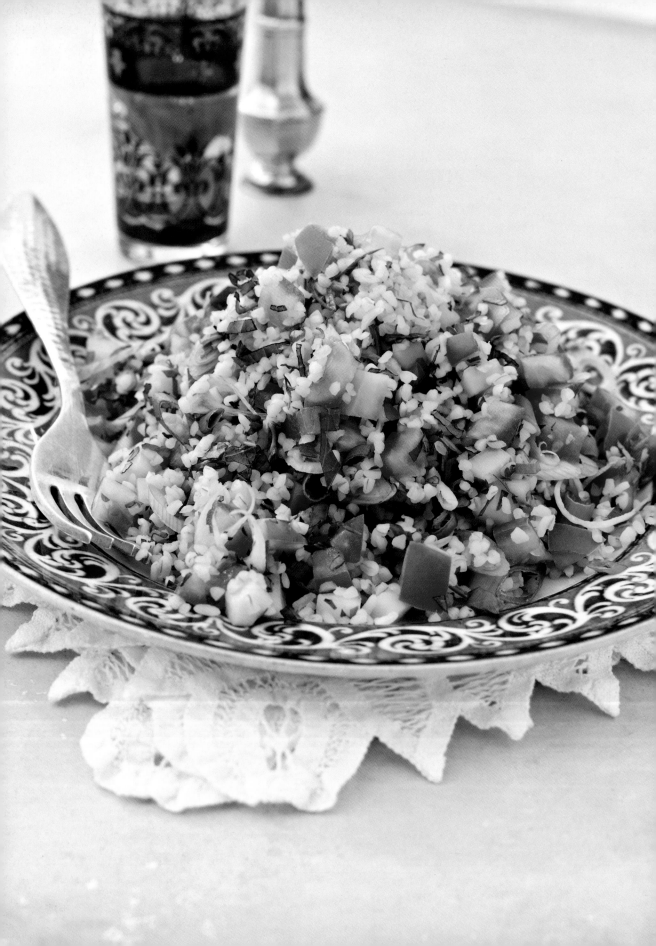

Moroccan bulgur wheat salad

SERVES 4

EASY Ⓥ ❄

Syns per serving
Extra Easy: Free
Green: Free
Original: 2½

Preparation time 10 minutes plus soaking

50g/2oz raw bulgur wheat
1 bunch spring onions, trimmed and finely chopped
3 tomatoes, skinned and chopped
¼ cucumber, peeled and diced
a large bunch of flat-leaf parsley, finely chopped
a few mint sprigs, chopped
salt and freshly ground black pepper
4 tbsp lemon juice

This healthy wholegrain salad is popular throughout the Mediterranean and is traditionally made with olive oil, but we have used lemon juice instead.

Put the bulgur wheat in a sieve and wash under cold running water, then transfer to a large bowl and cover with fresh cold water. Leave to soak for 30 minutes, then drain and squeeze dry.

Mix the bulgur wheat with the spring onions, tomatoes, cucumber, parsley and mint. Season well and stir in the lemon juice. Serve immediately.

Falafel

SERVES 6

WORTH THE EFFORT Ⓥ ✳

Syns per serving
Extra Easy: Free
Green: Free
Original: 6

Preparation time 1 hour plus chilling
Cooking time 12–15 minutes

225g/8oz dried chickpeas
1 onion, peeled and finely chopped
2 garlic cloves, peeled and crushed
2 eggs, beaten
1 tsp ground cumin
1 tsp ground coriander
1 small red chilli, deseeded and finely chopped
1 tbsp chopped coriander
2 tbsp chopped flat-leaf parsley
¼ tsp baking powder
salt and freshly ground black pepper
low calorie cooking spray

TO SERVE
fat free natural yogurt flavoured with chopped mint and red chilli

These spicy little snacks are sold by street vendors throughout northern Africa. The falafel are usually deep-fried for a really crisp finish, but they taste just as good baked in the oven.

Put the chickpeas in a large saucepan of water, boil for 45 minutes and drain well. Transfer to a food processor and add the onion, garlic, eggs, cumin, ground coriander, chilli and herbs. Process until you have a thick, smooth purée. Add the baking powder and seasoning and stir well. Transfer to a bowl and chill for 1 hour or overnight, if time permits.

When you are ready to cook the falafel, preheat the oven to 220°C/Gas 7 and spray a baking sheet with low calorie cooking spray. Take small pieces of the puréed chickpea mixture and form into little balls between your hands then flatten them out slightly and arrange them on the prepared baking sheet.

Cook the falafel in the oven for 12–15 minutes, until crisp and golden. Serve immediately with a bowl of the yogurt dip.

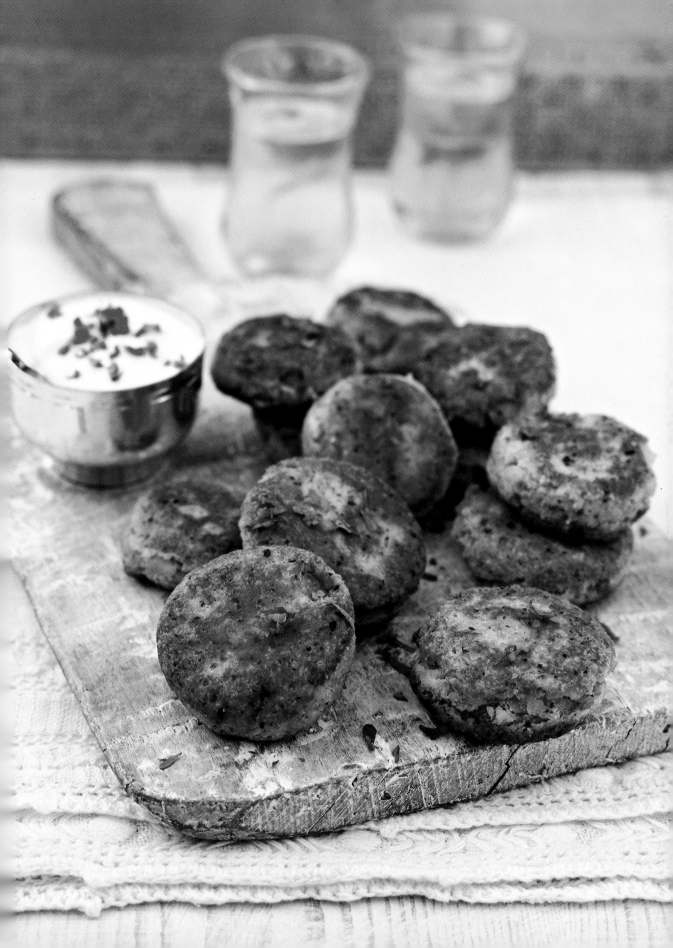

Warm herbed couscous salad

SERVES 4

EASY Ⓥ

Syns per serving
Extra Easy: ½
Green: ½
Original: 20½

Preparation time 10–12 minutes
Cooking time under 10 minutes

300g/11oz dried couscous
salt and freshly ground black pepper
low calorie cooking spray
2 tsp ground ginger
2 tsp ground cumin
1 tsp ground cinnamon
1 red onion, peeled, halved
and thinly sliced
1 red pepper, deseeded and chopped
400g can chickpeas, drained
and rinsed
300g/11oz cherry tomatoes, halved
a small handful of coriander,
roughly chopped
a small handful of mint,
roughly chopped
juice of 1 orange

This salad is perfect for easy entertaining – it takes very little time to prepare and uses everyday ingredients. For a variation, toss some grilled prawns or chicken into the finished dish.

Place the couscous in a wide, heatproof bowl, season well and pour over enough boiling water to just cover the grains. Cover tightly and allow to stand for 10–12 minutes.

Meanwhile, spray a large non-stick frying pan with low calorie cooking spray and place over a medium heat. Add the spices, onion, pepper and chickpeas and stir-fry for 4–5 minutes.

Turn the heat to high and add 60ml/2fl oz of hot water and the cherry tomatoes. Stir-fry for 2–3 minutes or until the vegetables are softened, but still retain a bite.

Fluff up the couscous grains with a fork and add to the pan together with the herbs and orange juice. Check the seasoning, toss to mix well and serve immediately in warmed bowls.

Harira

SERVES 4

EASY Ⓥ

Syns per serving
Extra Easy: Free
Green: Free
Original: 13½

Preparation time 15 minutes plus
overnight soaking
Cooking time 2½–3 hours

175g/6oz dried chickpeas
1 onion, peeled and chopped
1 celery stick, trimmed and chopped
1.5 litres/2½ pints vegetable stock
1 tsp turmeric
1 tsp paprika
1 tsp ground cinnamon
450g/1lb tomatoes, skinned
and chopped
110g/4oz red split lentils
50g/2oz dried vermicelli pasta
salt and freshly ground black pepper
2 tbsp chopped flat-leaf parsley
2 tbsp chopped coriander

TO SERVE
lemon wedges
harissa paste (optional)

This soup is always made in Morocco and other North African Mahgreb countries during the festival of Ramadan. It is eaten at sunset when the daily fast comes to an end. For a fiery hot soup stir in a little harissa pasta just before serving.

Put the chickpeas in a bowl and cover with cold water. Leave to soak overnight. Drain and rinse under cold running water, then set aside.

Put the onion and celery in a large saucepan with 300ml/½ pint of the stock. Cover the pan and bring to the boil. Boil for 5–10 minutes, then reduce the heat, uncover and simmer for 25–30 minutes, until the vegetables are tender, golden and syrupy.

Stir in the spices and cook gently for 2 minutes, then add the tomatoes and lentils along with the drained chickpeas. Cook gently, stirring occasionally, for 5 minutes.

Add the remaining stock and simmer for 1½–2 hours, until the chickpeas are cooked and tender.

Add the vermicelli and simmer gently for 15 minutes. Just before serving, check the seasoning, then stir in the herbs.

Serve the soup with lemon wedges and a little bowl of harissa paste, if using.

Harissa prawns

Harissa is a Moroccan spice paste, used widely for flavouring meat and fish dishes. It can be bought ready made but here we make it from scratch for these tasty prawn skewers.

SERVES 4

EASY ❄ (only if prawns are fresh)

Syns per serving
Extra Easy: Free
Original: Free
Green: 7

Preparation time 30 minutes
Cooking time under 10 minutes

24 raw tiger or king prawns, peeled but with tails left on
20 bay leaves

FOR THE HARISSA PASTE
50g/2oz long red chillies, deseeded
sea salt
3 heaped tsp caraway seeds, ground
3 heaped tsp cumin seeds, ground
2 tsp cumin seeds, ground
4 garlic cloves, peeled
100g/3½oz roasted and peeled red pepper
4 tsp passata
4 tsp red wine vinegar
juice of 2 lemons
2 level tsp smoked paprika

TO SERVE
a crisp green salad
fat free natural yogurt

First make the harissa paste. Blend the chillies in a food processor with a pinch of sea salt, half of each of the spice seeds and the garlic until smooth.

Add the pepper, the rest of the spices, the passata and vinegar, and blend again until very smooth. Transfer to a mixing bowl.

Add the lemon juice, sprinkle with the paprika and stir in. Season with more salt, if necessary, to balance out the vinegar.

Tip the prawns into the harissa paste and toss to coat well. Thread six prawns onto each of four metal skewers or presoaked wooden skewers, alternating the prawns with a bay leaf.

Heat a griddle pan and when smoking hot add the prawn skewers and cook for about 5 minutes, basting occasionally with the harissa paste, and turning at least once, until the prawns turn pink and are cooked through. Serve with a crisp green salad and some cooling yogurt to dip the prawns into.

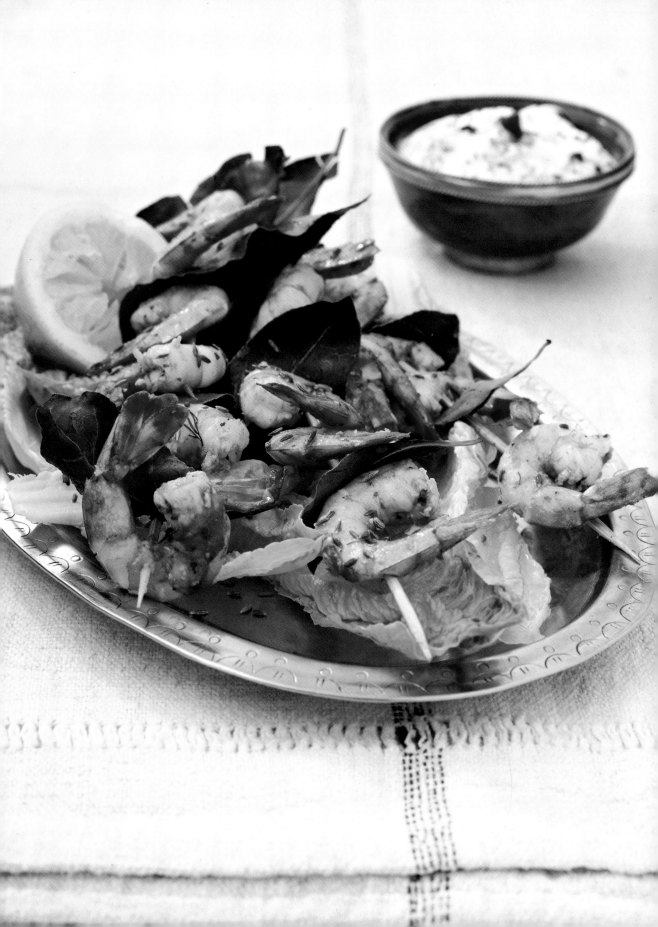

Moroccan grilled sardines

SERVES 4

REALLY EASY

Syns per serving
Extra Easy: Free
Original: Free
Green: 49½

Preparation time 10 minutes
Cooking time 10 minutes

12 large sardines, gutted and cleaned
2 tbsp ready-made harissa paste or
Moroccan spice blend
finely grated zest and juice of 2 lemons
salt and freshly ground black pepper

TO SERVE
lemon wedges

We've used ready-made harissa paste for this tasty fish dish but you could make your own using the recipe from Harissa Prawns (page 120).

Preheat the grill to its highest setting. Rinse the sardines and pat them dry with kitchen paper. Make three deep cuts on both sides of each fish with a sharp knife.

Mix the harissa paste or Moroccan spice blend with the lemon zest and juice to make a thin paste and rub into both sides of the sardines.

Put the sardines on a non-stick baking sheet and grill them for 3–4 minutes on each side, depending on how big they are. To check if they're done, gently pull a back fin – it will come out easily if the sardine is cooked. Season and serve with lemon wedges to squeeze over.

Chermoula fish skewers

SERVES 4

EASY

Syns per serving
Extra Easy: Free
Original: Free
Green: 9

Preparation time 15 minutes
plus marinating
Cooking time 6–8 minutes

Chermoula is a Moroccan spice mix made with cumin, coriander, garlic, paprika and lemon juice and can be used to marinate fish or chicken before grilling or cooking on the barbecue.

FOR THE CHERMOULA MARINADE
2 tbsp sweet paprika
3 tbsp finely chopped coriander
1 tsp ground coriander
2 tsp roughly ground cumin seeds
8 garlic cloves, peeled and crushed
juice of 2 lemons
1 small red onion, peeled and
very finely chopped
1 tsp cayenne pepper
2 tbsp chopped flat-leaf parsley
salt and freshly ground black pepper

FOR THE FISH SKEWERS
900g/2lb skinless and boneless thick
cod fillets, cut into bite-sized pieces
1 green pepper, deseeded and
cut into bite-sized pieces
1 red pepper, deseeded and
cut into bite-sized pieces
1 yellow pepper, deseeded and
cut into bite-sized pieces

TO SERVE
a few coriander and mint sprigs
lime or lemon wedges

To make the chermoula marinade, put all the ingredients in a shallow ceramic dish and stir until smooth. Season well. Add the cod to the marinade and turn until the pieces are coated all over. Cover and chill for 1–2 hours, or overnight if time permits.

When you are ready to eat the kebabs, preheat the grill to medium or prepare the barbecue. Thread the cod pieces onto 12 metal skewers or presoaked wooden skewers, alternating them with the pieces of pepper. Place under the grill or on the barbecue in a single layer and cook for 2–3 minutes on each side, or until the fish is just cooked through. Garnish with coriander and mint sprigs and serve immediately with lime or lemon wedges.

Chicken tagine

SERVES 4

EASY ✻

Syns per serving
Extra Easy: Free
Original: Free
Green: 14

Preparation time 25 minutes
Cooking time 1 hour 10 minutes

2 tsp saffron threads
250ml/9fl oz boiling hot chicken stock
2 large onions, peeled and
finely chopped
1 tsp ground ginger
1 tsp ground cumin
3 garlic cloves, peeled and finely sliced
1kg/2lb 4oz skinless and boneless
chicken thighs, cut into large
bite-sized pieces
1 tsp black peppercorns, crushed
6 small preserved lemons, quartered,
or 2 larger ones, chopped
6 tbsp roughly chopped coriander
6 tbsp roughly chopped flat-leaf
parsley

Preserved lemons are used extensively in Middle Eastern and North African cooking. Whole lemons, or sometimes lemon slices, are packed in jars with salt. They are available from delicatessens or some supermarkets.

Add the saffron threads to the stock and leave to infuse for 15 minutes.

Place the onions, stock, ginger, cumin and garlic in a heavy-based, flameproof lidded casserole dish and bring to the boil.

Add the chicken, peppercorns and lemons and bring back to a simmer, then cover and cook on a very gentle heat for about 1 hour, or until the chicken is very tender. Remove from the heat and add the coriander and parsley just before serving.

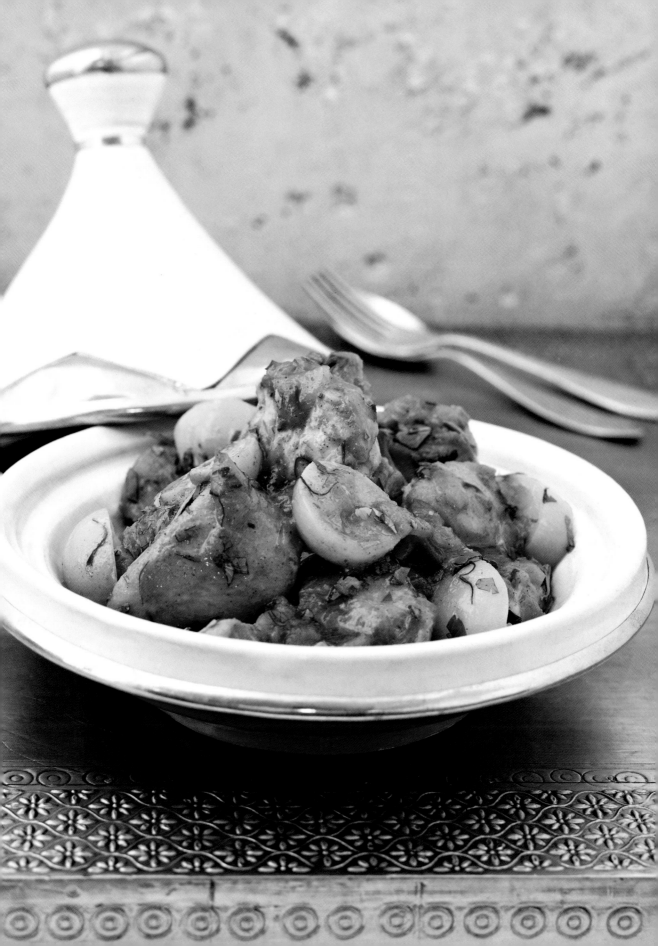

Lamb tagine

SERVES 4

EASY ❋

Syns per serving
Extra Easy: 2½
Original: 2½
Green: 11

Preparation time 15 minutes
Cooking time 2 hours

1 large onion, peeled and chopped
2 green peppers, deseeded
and chopped
2 garlic cloves, peeled and crushed
600ml/1 pint lamb stock
1 tsp ground ginger
2 tsp ground cinnamon
450g/1lb lean lamb, cut into cubes
a large pinch of saffron threads
110g/4oz semi-dried apricots, chopped
salt and freshly ground black pepper
1 tbsp lemon juice
2 tbsp chopped flat-leaf parsley

Spicy stews of meat and fresh and dried fruit are common in northern Africa and are often served at celebrations and on festive occasions. This is delicious served with rice or couscous.

Put the onion, peppers, garlic and half the stock in a large saucepan, cover and bring to the boil. Boil for 10 minutes until the vegetables are softened, then reduce the heat, uncover the pan and simmer for 20–30 minutes, until the onions are golden, tender and syrupy.

Stir in the ginger, cinnamon and lamb cubes, and cook for 4–5 minutes, turning the lamb occasionally, until browned all over. Add the remaining stock and the saffron and cover the pan. Leave to simmer gently for 1 hour, adding more stock if necessary.

Add the apricots, season and simmer for a further 15 minutes until the apricots are tender.

Check the seasoning and stir in the lemon juice. If the tagine has too much liquid, boil hard for a few minutes to reduce the sauce to a thicker consistency. Sprinkle with the parsley and serve.

Moroccan lamb chops with cucumber salad and chickpea purée

SERVES 4

EASY ✳

Syns per serving
Extra Easy: Free
Green: 5½
Original: 6

Preparation time 15 minutes
Cooking time 10–12 minutes

FOR THE CUCUMBER SALAD
150g/5oz fat free natural yogurt
½ cucumber, diced
salt and freshly ground black pepper

FOR THE CHICKPEA PURÉE
400g can chickpeas, drained and rinsed
1 garlic clove, peeled and crushed
1 tsp ground coriander
1 tsp ground cumin
1 tbsp chopped flat-leaf parsley

FOR THE LAMB
4 lean lamb chops
2 tsp ground paprika
½ small onion, peeled and grated

This recipe is loosely based on the Moroccan way of cooking and serving lamb, where grated onion and hot spices are sprinkled on to the grilled meat.

First make the cucumber salad. Mix the yogurt with the diced cucumber and season to taste. Chill in the fridge until required.

To make the chickpea purée, blend the chickpeas, garlic, spices and parsley with an electric hand-held blender or in a food processor until mushy. If the purée is too thick, thin it with a little water. Season to taste and set aside in a cool place.

When ready to cook, preheat the grill to hot or prepare the barbecue. Cook the lamb chops under the grill in a ridged grill pan or on the barbecue until cooked and crisp outside but still juicy inside (this will take 3–4 minutes each side for pink, and 5-6 minutes for well done). Season and sprinkle with the paprika and onion. Serve immediately with the cucumber salad and chickpea purée.

Orange, mint and pomegranate salad

SERVES 4

REALLY EASY (V)

Syns per serving
Extra Easy: ½
Original: ½
Green: ½

Preparation time 20 minutes

5–6 large sweet oranges
1 large pomegranate, seeds and any juices removed and reserved
8 tbsp freshly squeezed orange juice
1 tbsp lemon juice
freshly ground black pepper
6 tbsp roughly chopped mint

Jewel-like pomegranate seeds perfectly complement the sweet orange segments in this colourful and refreshing Moroccan fruit salad.

Use a sharp knife to take a slice off the top and bottom of each orange, then place the fruit on a chopping board and carefully cut away the skin and pith, following the curve of the orange. Cut the fruit into horizontal slices, reserving any juice for the dressing.

Arrange the orange slices on a large serving plate and sprinkle over the pomegranate seeds.

To make the dressing, whisk together the orange and lemon juice and any reserved pomegranate juice. Season to taste with black pepper and drizzle over the salad. Scatter over the chopped mint and serve.

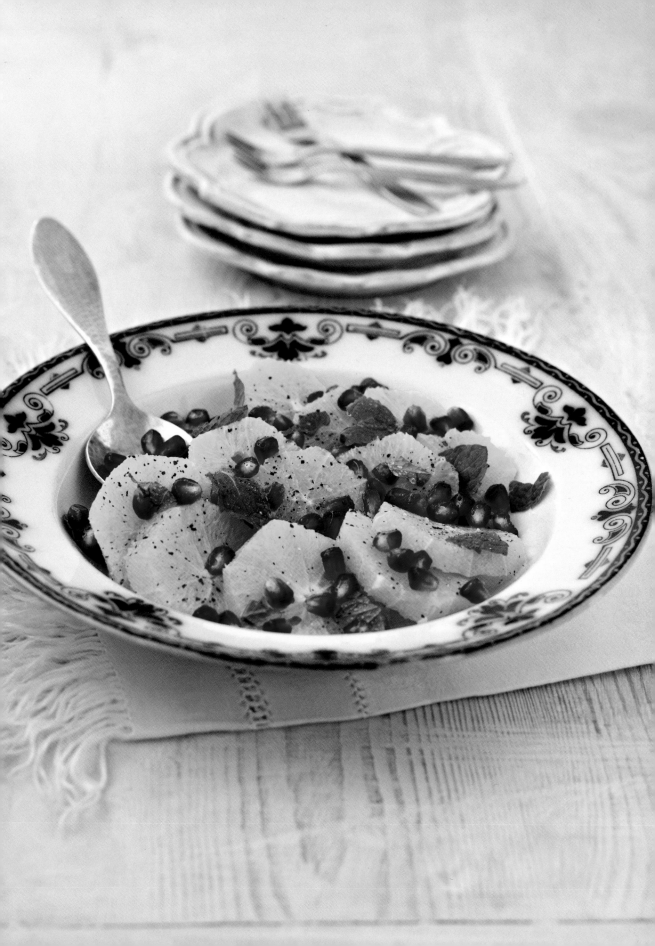

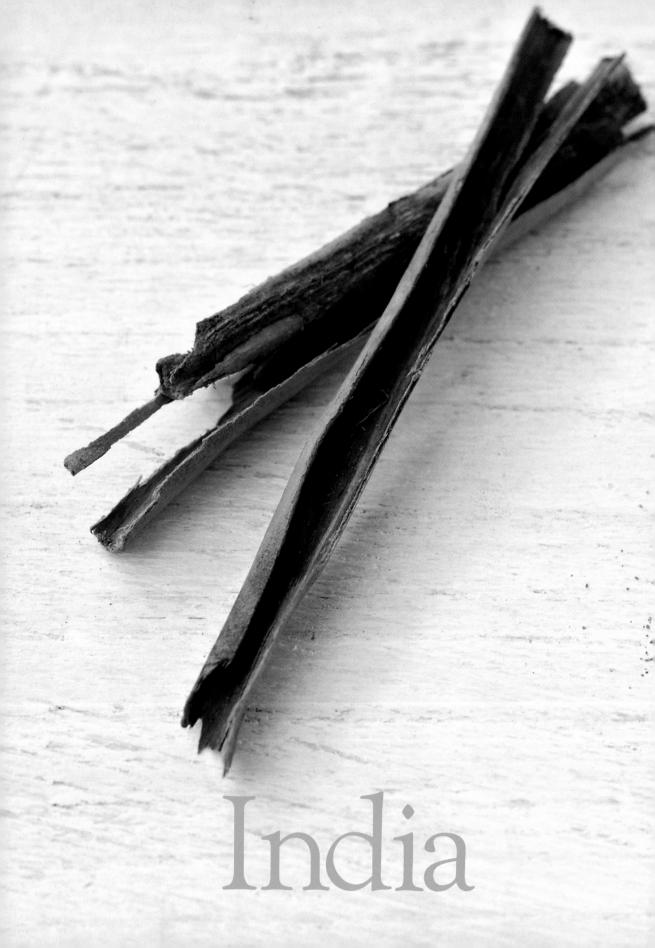

India

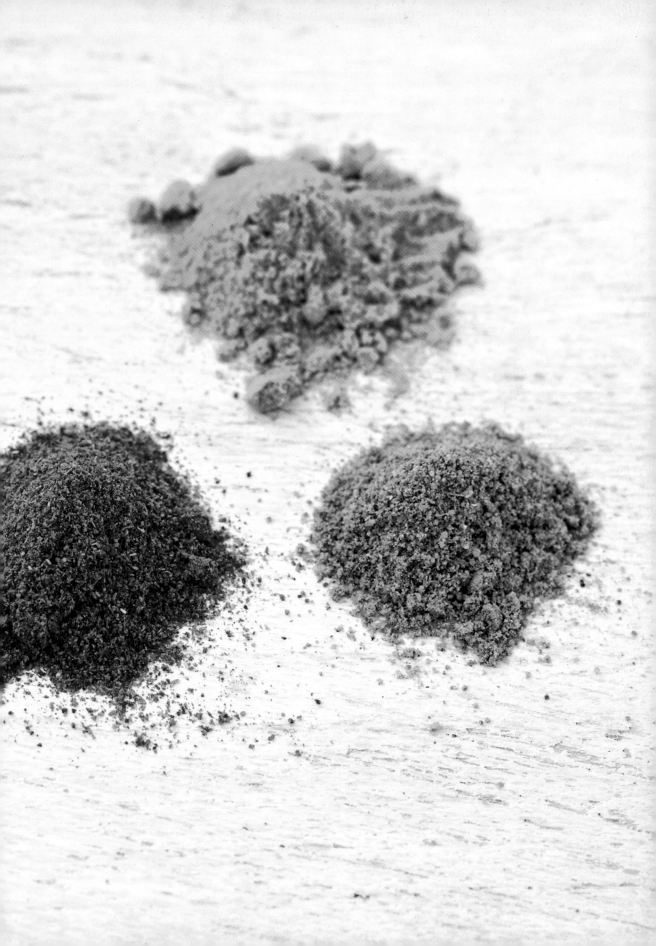

Aloo gobi

In this lightly spiced dish potatoes and cauliflower are cooked with peas and cherry tomatoes. This is delicious served with steamed basmati rice.

Syns per serving
Extra Easy: Free
Green: Free
Original: 5

Preparation time 20 minutes
Cooking time under 25 minutes

4 medium potatoes, peeled and cut into 1.5cm/½in cubes
low calorie cooking spray
1 tsp black mustard seeds
1 tsp cumin seeds
1 tsp ground coriander
1 tsp ground cumin
½ tsp turmeric
¼ tsp ground cloves
¼ tsp ground ginger
1 onion, peeled, halved and sliced
½ cauliflower, cut into florets
2 bay leaves
10 cherry tomatoes, halved
100g/3½oz frozen peas
1 tbsp lemon juice

Boil the potatoes in lightly salted water for about 5–6 minutes, or until just barely tender. Remove from the heat and drain.

Spray a wok or deep non-stick lidded frying pan with low calorie cooking spray and place over a medium heat. Add the spices and stir-fry for about 30 seconds, then add the onion, cauliflower, bay leaves, tomatoes, peas and potatoes. Allow the vegetables to cook for 4–5 minutes, then add the lemon juice and 300ml/11fl oz of water.

Cover and cook for another 6–8 minutes, or until the vegetables are tender. Remove from the heat and serve immediately.

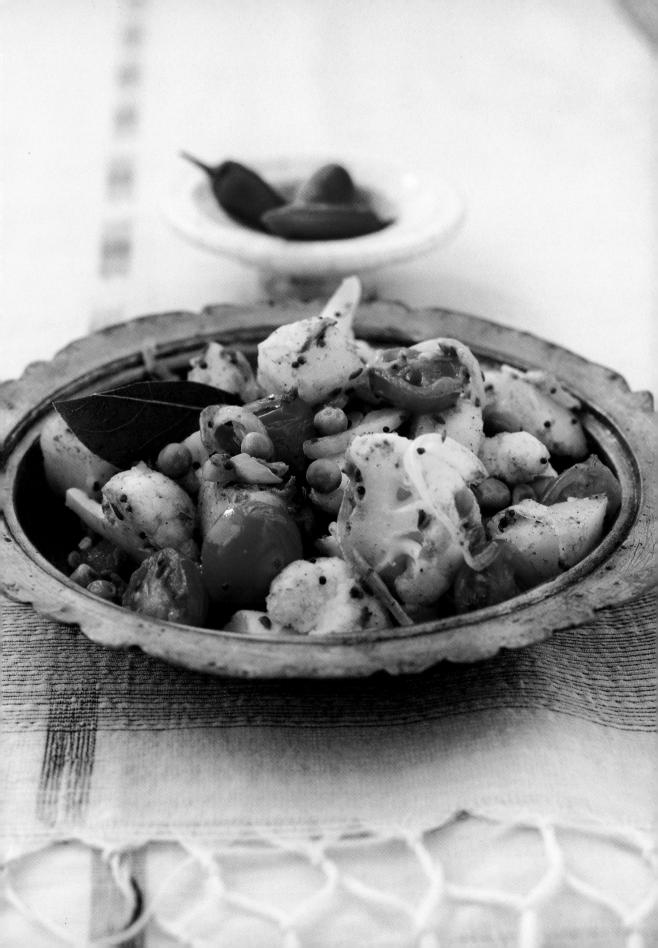

Tarka dal

SERVES 4

WORTH THE EFFORT (V) (❄)

Syns per serving
Extra Easy: Free
Green: Free
Original: 9½

Preparation time 15 minutes
Cooking time 30–35 minutes

FOR THE DAL
250g/9oz dried red split lentils
1 tsp turmeric
4 tomatoes, roughly chopped
salt and freshly ground black pepper
6–8 tbsp finely chopped coriander

FOR THE TARKA
low calorie cooking spray
2 tsp black mustard seeds
3 tsp cumin seeds
2 garlic cloves, peeled and
very thinly sliced
2 tsp very finely chopped root ginger
6–8 curry leaves
1 whole dried red chilli
2 tsp ground cumin
2 tsp ground coriander

Here is the ultimate basic Indian comfort food! In this recipe, the cooked lentils are given a final seasoning with spices to add even more flavour to the dish.

Place the lentils in a large fine-mesh sieve and run cold water over them until the water runs clear. Drain well and place in a heavy-based saucepan with 1 litre/1¾ pints of water. Bring to the boil over a high heat and skim away any scum that comes to the surface. Reduce the heat to medium and continue to cook for 20–25 minutes or until the lentils have softened.

Remove from the heat and, using an electric hand-held blender or whisk, blend until smooth. Return to the heat and stir in the turmeric and tomatoes. Bring to the boil, season and stir in the coriander.

Meanwhile, make the tarka. Spray a large non-stick frying pan with low calorie cooking spray. When hot, add all the tarka ingredients and stir-fry for 1–2 minutes until the spices darken and their aroma is released.

Remove from the heat and spoon over the cooked dal. Stir and serve immediately.

Indian potatoes with whole spices

SERVES 4

EASY Ⓥ ⁂

Syns per serving
Extra Easy: Free
Green: Free
Original: 4½

Preparation time 5 minutes
Cooking time 30–35 minutes

450g/1lb potatoes, peeled and
thickly sliced
low calorie cooking spray
1 onion, peeled and thinly
sliced into rings
1 red chilli, deseeded and
finely chopped
½ tsp turmeric
½ tsp garam masala
¼ tsp cumin seeds
1 cinnamon stick
8 green cardamom pods
salt and freshly ground black pepper
3 tbsp chopped coriander

TO SERVE
fat free natural yogurt (optional)

Slices of potato cooked with aromatic spices are always a welcome accompaniment. This recipe goes really well with cold roast meats, such as chicken, turkey, lamb or beef.

Cook the potatoes in a large saucepan of lightly salted boiling water for 10–15 minutes or until just tender. Drain and keep warm.

Spray a large non-stick frying pan with low calorie cooking spray and place over a medium heat. Add the onion and cook for about 5 minutes, until softened and golden brown. Add the chilli and all the spices and continue cooking gently for 2–3 minutes to allow the spices to release their aroma.

Add the potatoes, cover the pan and cook over a low heat for about 10 minutes, turning the potatoes occasionally. Season, if necessary, and sprinkle with the coriander.

Eat the potatoes hot accompanied with a bowl of cooling yogurt, if wished.

Chickpea and spinach curry

SERVES 4

EASY Ⓥ ❄

Syns per serving
Extra Easy: Free
Green: Free
Original: 9½

Preparation time 10 minutes
Cooking time 25 minutes

low calorie cooking spray
2 onions, peeled and thinly sliced
2 garlic cloves, peeled and crushed
2.5cm/1in piece root ginger, peeled and grated
1 tsp turmeric
1 tsp garam masala
1 tsp coriander seeds
1 tsp ground coriander
1 tsp cumin seeds
1–2 red chillies, deseeded and chopped
400g can chopped tomatoes
450g/1lb spinach leaves, trimmed
600g/1lb 6oz canned chickpeas, drained and rinsed
salt and freshly ground black pepper
2 tbsp chopped coriander or mint

TO SERVE
boiled rice

In India, chickpeas are known as 'chhole' and they are often added to vegetable curries – they are a great source of fibre and when cooked have a lovely nutty flavour.

Spray a large saucepan with low calorie cooking spray and place over a medium heat. Add the onions, garlic and ginger and cook for about 5 minutes, until softened and golden.

Add the spices and chillies, stir well and cook gently for about 3 minutes to allow the spices to release their aroma. Then stir in the tomatoes and spinach and reduce the heat to a bare simmer. Simmer gently for a further 5 minutes and, finally, add the chickpeas.

Continue simmering for 5–10 minutes, until the spinach has wilted and the tomato liquid has reduced. Season and stir in the coriander or mint. Serve immediately with some plain boiled rice.

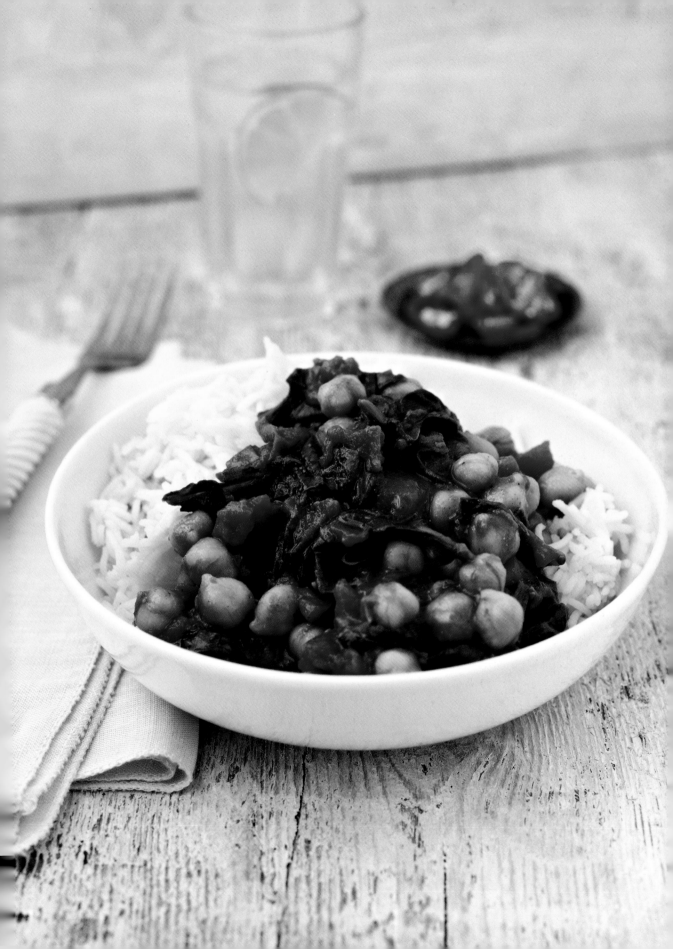

Spiced Indian beans

SERVES 4

WORTH THE EFFORT Ⓥ ❋

Syns per serving
Extra Easy: Free
Green: Free
Original: 5

Preparation time 15 minutes
Cooking time 40 minutes

low calorie cooking spray
2 onions, peeled and finely chopped
2 garlic cloves, peeled and chopped
2.5cm/1in piece root ginger,
peeled and finely chopped
1 green chilli, deseeded and chopped
½ tsp turmeric
1 tsp crushed coriander seeds
½ tsp cumin seeds
4 tomatoes, skinned and quartered
300ml/½ pint vegetable stock
400g can kidney beans, drained and
rinsed
175g/6oz spinach leaves, trimmed and
shredded
225g/8oz fat free natural yogurt
salt and freshly ground black pepper
small bunch of coriander, chopped

TO SERVE
boiled rice

In this creamy Indian dish, cooked red kidney beans are added to a spiced tomato and yogurt sauce.

Spray a large non-stick frying pan with low calorie cooking spray and place over a medium heat. Add the onions, garlic and ginger and cook for 5 minutes, until softened. Add the chilli, turmeric, coriander and cumin seeds and cook gently for 2–3 minutes, stirring occasionally, to allow the spices to release their aroma.

Add the tomatoes, stock and kidney beans. Simmer over a low heat for about 25 minutes. Remove some of the beans and mash coarsely, then return them to the sauce.

Stir in the spinach and yogurt and continue cooking over a low heat for 5 minutes, until the spinach wilts and is cooked.

Season and stir in the coriander. Serve immediately with boiled rice.

Spicy cabbage and tomatoes

SERVES 4

EASY Ⓥ

Syns per serving
Extra Easy: Free
Original: Free
Green: Free

Preparation time 20 minutes
Cooking time 45–50 minutes

900g/2lb cabbage
2 onions, peeled and thinly sliced
2 garlic cloves, peeled and crushed
300ml/½ pint vegetable stock
2.5cm/1in piece root ginger, peeled and sliced
1 tsp chilli powder
2 tsp turmeric
1 tsp ground coriander
1 tsp cumin seeds
½ tsp mustard seeds
salt and freshly ground black pepper
350g/12oz tomatoes, skinned and roughly chopped

Fresh cabbage is eaten throughout India. In this delicious dish, it is flavoured with a selection of aromatic spices and then cooked with tomatoes until it is just tender. It would be a great accompaniment to grilled meats or fluffy boiled rice.

Wash the cabbage thoroughly under cold running water then pat dry with kitchen paper. Cut out any thick stems and slice the leaves into thin strips. Set aside.

Put the onions, garlic and stock in a large, heavy-based saucepan. Cover and bring to the boil. Boil for 10 minutes, then uncover and cook gently over a low heat for 20 minutes, until the onions are tender, golden and syrupy.

Stir in the ginger, chilli powder, turmeric, coriander and cumin and mustard seeds. Cook over a gentle heat for about 5 minutes.

Add the cabbage and toss gently to coat it with the spicy onion mixture. Season well and add the tomatoes. If the mixture is dry, add a little more stock or boiling water.

Simmer gently for 5–10 minutes, until the cabbage is tender and cooked but still quite firm. Serve immediately.

Vegetable curry

SERVES 4

EASY Ⓥ ❄

Syns per serving
Extra Easy: Free
Original: Free
Green: Free

Preparation time 15–20 minutes
Cooking time about 1 hour

FOR THE SPICE MIXTURE
2 tbsp cumin seeds
1 tbsp coriander seeds
1 tbsp cardamom seeds
1 tsp mustard seeds
4 cloves

FOR THE CURRY
2 onions, peeled and sliced
2 garlic cloves, peeled and crushed
600ml/1 pint vegetable stock
1 red chilli, deseeded and finely
chopped
2.5cm/1in piece root ginger, peeled and
chopped
1 tsp turmeric
110g/4oz button mushrooms
1 aubergine, cubed
110g/4oz cauliflower florets
110g/4oz broccoli florets
150g/5oz fat free natural yogurt
salt and freshly ground black pepper
2 tbsp chopped coriander

The addition of fat free natural yogurt gives this curry a marvellous creamy texture. Serve with refreshing sliced tomato, cucumber and banana together with plain boiled rice.

To make the spice mixture, grind all the spices together in an electric grinder or with a pestle and mortar.

To make the curry, put the onions, garlic and half the stock in a heavy-based saucepan, cover and bring to the boil for 5–10 minutes. Then uncover and simmer for 20–30 minutes, until the onions are tender, golden and syrupy.

Add the chilli, ginger, turmeric and ground spice mixture and cook gently for 2–3 minutes to allow the spices to release their aroma. Then add the mushrooms, aubergine and cauliflower along with the remaining stock. Cover the pan and simmer for about 20 minutes.

Meanwhile, cook the broccoli separately in lightly salted boiling water until it just tender and still a lovely bright green, then drain and add to the curry. Remove from the heat and stir in the yogurt.

Check the seasoning and serve the curry immediately, scattered with the coriander.

Vegetable biryani

SERVES 4

WORTH THE EFFORT Ⓥ ❄

Syns per serving
Extra Easy: 3
Green: 3
Original: 13

Preparation time 15 minutes
Cooking time 1–1¼ hours

1 large onion, peeled and finely chopped
1 small aubergine, cubed
2 garlic cloves, peeled and crushed
900ml/1½ pints vegetable stock
1 tsp ground coriander
½ tsp ground cumin
¼ tsp ground turmeric
4 cloves
4 green cardamom pods
2.5cm/1in piece cinnamon stick
1 red chilli, deseeded and finely chopped
2.5cm/1in piece root ginger, peeled and finely chopped
225g/8oz dried rice
2 carrots, peeled and sliced
2 courgettes, sliced
1 small cauliflower, divided into florets
110g/4oz tiny button mushrooms
15g/½oz sultanas
salt and freshly ground black pepper
2 tbsp flaked almonds, toasted

Serve this biryani with a Syn-free raita made from fat free natural yogurt mixed with diced cucumber and chopped fresh mint.

Put the onion, aubergine, garlic and one-third of the stock in a large saucepan, cover and bring to the boil. Boil for 5–10 minutes, then uncover the pan, reduce the heat and simmer for about 20 minutes, until the vegetables are tender and syrupy.

Add all the spices, chilli and ginger and stir well. Cook gently for 2 minutes to allow the aroma of the spices to be released then add the rice. Cook over a very low heat, stirring occasionally, for 2–3 minutes, until all the grains are coated.

Add the carrots, courgettes, cauliflower, mushrooms and the remaining stock. Bring to the boil, then reduce the heat and simmer gently for 25–30 minutes, until the vegetables are tender, the rice is cooked, and the liquid has been absorbed. Check the biryani occasionally, adding more water if necessary.

Remove the cinnamon stick, add the sultanas and season. Sprinkle with the almonds and serve.

Tandoori fish kebabs

Succulent pieces of monkfish are marinated in a blend of spices and yogurt and then quickly grilled. You could also barbecue these kebabs for that authentic tandoori flavour.

FOR THE MARINADE
350g/12oz fat free natural yogurt
2 tbsp finely grated onion
1 tbsp finely grated garlic
1 tbsp finely grated root ginger
juice of 2 limes
3 tbsp tandoori spice powder

FOR THE KEBABS
800g/1lb 12oz skinless monkfish fillets, cut into bite-sized pieces
4 red peppers, deseeded and cut into bite-sized pieces
salt and freshly ground black pepper

TO SERVE
chopped coriander and mint
fat free natural yogurt

Make the marinade by mixing together all the ingredients in a large bowl. Add the fish and peppers to the mixture, season well and toss to coat evenly. Cover and marinate in the fridge for 2–4 hours.

When ready to cook, preheat the grill to hot or prepare the barbecue. Thread the fish and pepper pieces alternately onto eight metal skewers, or presoaked wooden skewers, and cook under the grill or on the barbecue for 4–5 minutes on each side, or until the fish is just cooked through.

Garnish with coriander and mint and serve immediately with a bowl of yogurt.

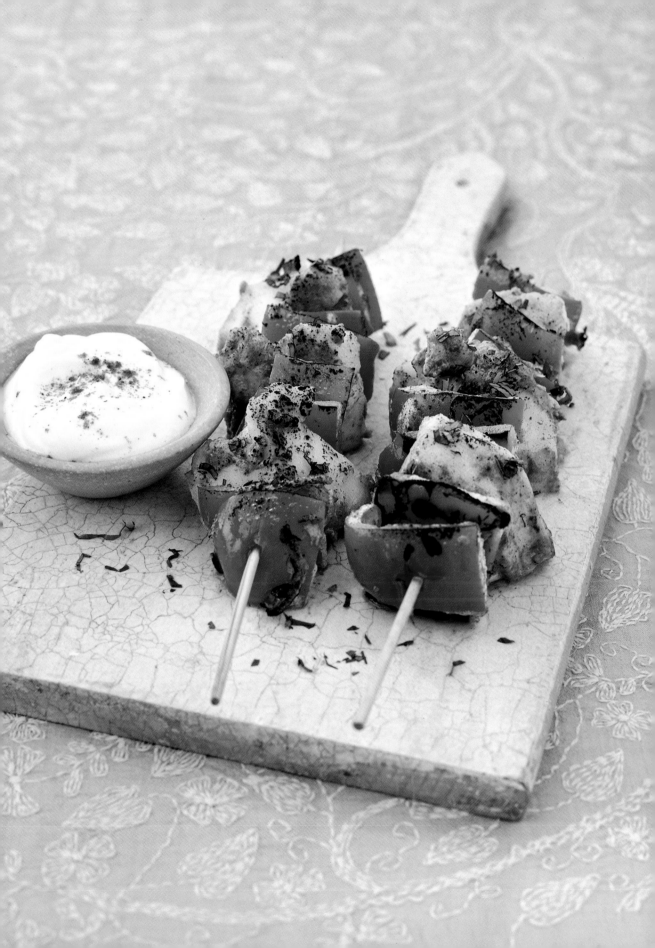

Goan prawn curry

SERVES 4

EASY ❄ (only if prawns are fresh)

Syns per serving
Extra Easy: 3
Original: 3
Green: 10½

Preparation time 10 minutes
Cooking time under 20 minutes

1 tsp chilli powder
1 tbsp paprika
1 tsp turmeric
4 garlic cloves, peeled and crushed
2 tsp finely grated root ginger
2 tbsp ground cumin
2 tbsp passata
¼ tsp artificial sweetener
2 tsp tamarind paste
200ml/7fl oz light coconut milk
800g/1lb 12oz raw tiger prawns, peeled
but with tails left on
salt and freshly ground black pepper

TO SERVE
a few coriander sprigs
steamed white rice (optional)

As a variation, use large chunks of salmon or any other firm-fleshed fish instead of prawns in this spicy coastal curry.

Place the chilli powder, paprika, turmeric, garlic, ginger, cumin, passata and sweetener in a saucepan and mix with 300ml/11fl oz of water until smooth. Place the pan over a high heat and bring to the boil. Cover, reduce the heat and simmer gently for 8–10 minutes.

Stir in the tamarind paste and coconut milk and bring back to the boil. Add the prawns and cook for 6–7 minutes or until they are cooked through and have turned pink.

Season well and garnish with coriander sprigs. Serve immediately, with steamed white rice (2 Syns per 25g/1oz cooked on Original), if desired.

Tandoori chicken

SERVES 4

EASY ✻

Syns per serving
Extra Easy: Free
Original: Free
Green: 5

Preparation time 20 minutes plus
standing and marinating
Cooking time 15–20 minutes

8 skinless chicken drumsticks
juice of 1 lemon
½ tsp salt

FOR THE MARINADE
1 onion, peeled and finely chopped
3 garlic cloves, peeled and crushed
2.5cm/1in piece root ginger,
peeled and chopped
½ red chilli, deseeded and chopped
1 tsp ground coriander seeds
1 tsp ground cumin
1 tsp ground black pepper
275g/10oz fat free natural yogurt
a few drops of red food colouring

TO SERVE
lime wedges

Traditionally, tandoori dishes are cooked in hot clay ovens. Although we have chosen to grill these spicy and succulent chicken drumsticks, you could bake them in the oven instead for about 20 minutes on 220°C/Gas 7.

Make two or three cuts in each chicken drumstick with a sharp knife, deep enough to nearly reach the bone. Place the chicken in a large dish and sprinkle with the lemon juice and salt. Rub the salt and lemon mixture into the cuts in the chicken and then leave in a cool place for 30 minutes.

Meanwhile, make the marinade. Put the onion, garlic, ginger and red chilli in a blender or food processor and blend until smooth. Add the ground spices and yogurt, and blend again. Lastly, stir in a few drops of red food colouring.

Pour the marinade over the chicken drumsticks, cover and chill for about 12 hours (or up to 24 hours, if wished).

When ready to cook, preheat the grill to hot or prepare the barbecue. Remove the chicken from the marinade and arrange the drumsticks in a single layer under the grill or on the barbecue. Cook for 15–20 minutes, turning frequently and brushing with any remaining marinade, until the drumsticks are thoroughly cooked inside and crisp and slightly charred on the outside. Serve immediately with lime wedges.

Chicken vindaloo

SERVES 4

WORTH THE EFFORT ✳

Syns per serving
Extra Easy: ½
Original: ½
Green: 9½

Preparation time 20 minutes
plus marinating
Cooking time 1¼ hours

This extremely hot dish is for chilli aficionados who love really spicy food. It originated in Goa on the coast of south-west India where several European countries fought to capture the local spice trade.

FOR THE VINDALOO PASTE
2 tsp cumin seeds
2 hot dried red chillies
1 tsp black peppercorns
1 tsp cardamom pods
1 tsp fenugreek seeds
1 tsp black mustard seeds
1 tsp ground cinnamon
1 tbsp white wine vinegar
½ tsp salt
1 tsp soft brown sugar

FOR THE CHICKEN
4 x 175g/6oz skinless chicken breast
fillets, cut into large chunks
2 onions, peeled and thinly sliced
6 garlic cloves, peeled and crushed
2.5cm/1in piece root ginger,
peeled and chopped
300ml/½ pint chicken stock
2 tsp turmeric
2 tomatoes, skinned and chopped

To make the vindaloo paste, put all the whole spices in a spice grinder or pestle and mortar and grind to a powder. Mix with the cinnamon, vinegar, salt and sugar.

Rub the paste all over the chicken pieces, then place the chicken in a bowl and leave to marinate for 1 hour.

Put the onions, garlic, ginger and stock in a large heavy-based saucepan, cover and bring to the boil. Boil for 10 minutes, then uncover the pan and simmer gently for 20 minutes, until the onions are tender and golden. Stir in the turmeric and cook for 2 minutes.

Add the chicken, tomatoes and 150ml/¼ pint of water. Bring to the boil, then reduce the heat and simmer for at least 45 minutes, until the chicken is cooked and the sauce is thickened. Serve immediately.

Special saffron rice

SERVES 4

EASY (V)(❋)

Syns per serving
Extra Easy: 3
Green: 3
Original: 13

Preparation time 10 minutes plus soaking
Cooking time 50–60 minutes

½ tsp saffron threads
2 large onions, peeled and sliced
225g/8oz dried Basmati rice
1 tsp cloves
4 cardamom pods
1 tsp turmeric
½ tsp salt
½ tsp ground black peppercorns
300ml/½ pint boiling water
2 tbsp flaked almonds
15g/½oz sultanas

Saffron is very expensive but well worth buying for this golden, delicately scented, rice dish. The golden-red saffron threads are the stigma of the saffron crocus.

Put the saffron threads in a bowl and add 1 tablespoon of boiling water. Leave to soak for 20 minutes.

Meanwhile, put the onions and 300ml/½ pint of water in large, heavy-based saucepan. Cover, bring to the boil, and boil for 10 minutes. Uncover the pan, reduce the heat and simmer for 20 minutes, or until the onions are soft, golden and syrupy.

Add the rice, cloves, cardamom, turmeric, salt and peppercorns. Cook gently over a low heat for 3 minutes then add the boiling water, the saffron and its soaking liquid, the almonds and sultanas.

Stir well, lower the heat and simmer gently for 15–20 minutes, until the rice is cooked and has absorbed the liquid. Check the rice from time to time, stirring and adding more water if necessary. Serve immediately.

Kofta curry

Koftas are spicy meatballs. Here they are cooked in a colourful yogurt sauce and are delicious served with the Special Saffron Rice (see page 147).

(see page 147)

SERVES 4

WORTH THE EFFORT ✽

Syns per serving
Extra Easy: Free
Original: Free
Green: 7½

Preparation time 25 minutes
Cooking time 1 hour

450g/1lb extra lean minced beef
1 onion, peeled and finely chopped
2 garlic cloves, peeled and crushed
1 tsp ground cumin
2 tsp ground coriander
1 tsp ground ginger
1 tsp turmeric
½ tsp chilli powder
2 tbsp chopped coriander
1 egg, beaten

FOR THE SAUCE
1 onion, peeled and finely chopped
3 garlic cloves, peeled and crushed
600ml/1 pint beef stock
1 tbsp chopped root ginger
4 cloves
4 cardamom pods
2.5cm/1in piece cinnamon stick
1 tsp ground cumin
1 tsp coriander seeds, ground
1 tsp turmeric
3 tomatoes, skinned and chopped
5 tbsp fat free natural yogurt

TO SERVE
chopped coriander

Put the minced beef in a bowl with the onion, garlic, spices and chopped coriander and mix in the egg. Divide into 16 equal portions and shape into small balls. Set aside in a cool place.

To make the sauce, put the onion, garlic and half the stock in a large saucepan, cover and bring to the boil. Boil for 10 minutes, uncover and simmer for 20 minutes, until the onions are tender and syrupy. Stir the spices into the onion mixture and cook gently for 2–3 minutes. Add the tomatoes and yogurt and stir in gently, over a low heat. Add the remaining stock and heat through until it reaches simmering point.

Add the meatballs, cover and simmer gently for about 25 minutes until cooked through. Stir occasionally to prevent the sauce sticking. If necessary, add more stock or water as the sauce will reduce considerably. Sprinkle with chopped coriander and serve with Special Saffron Rice, if wished.

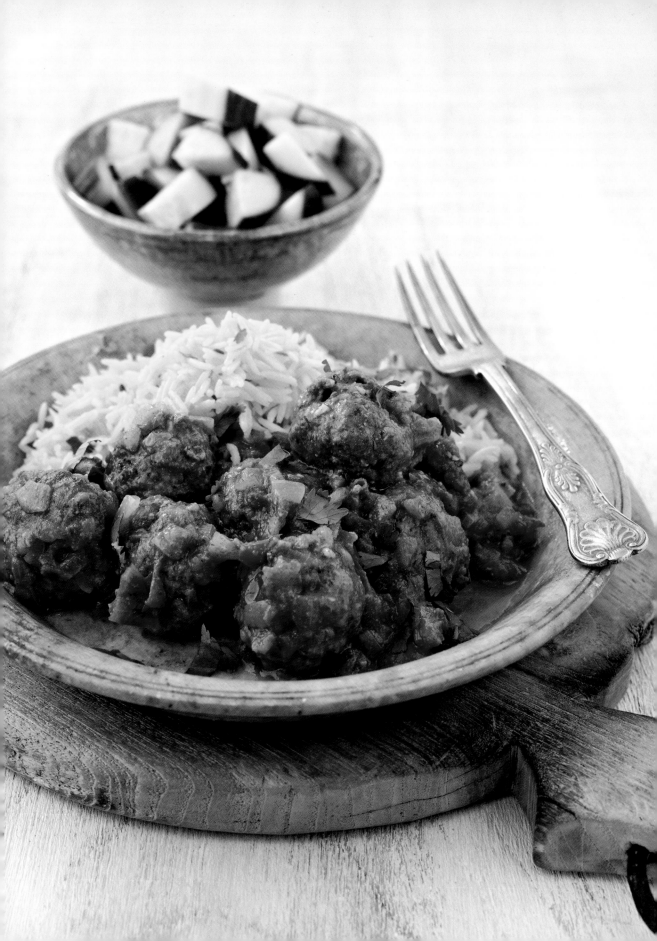

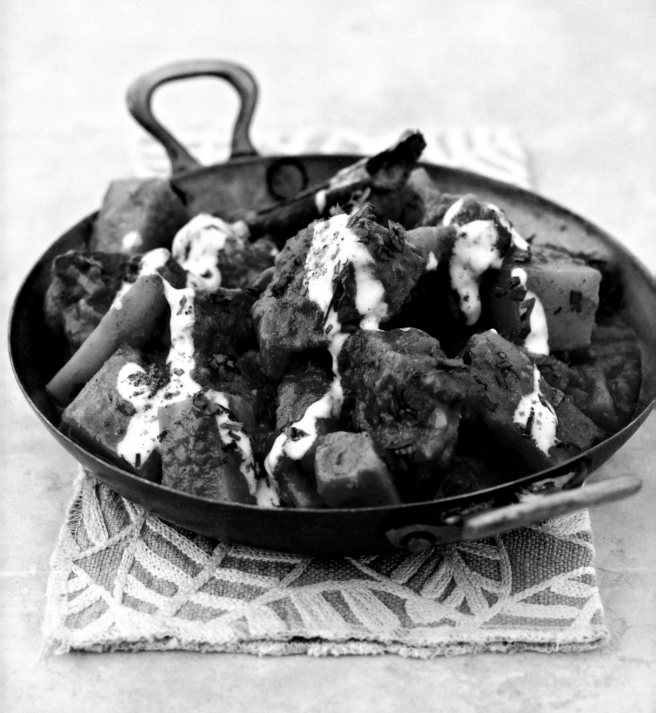

Lamb rogan josh

This rich, meaty lamb stew from northern India is flavoured with warming spices and cooked with chunks of carrot and swede.

SERVES 4

EASY ❄

Syns per serving
Extra Easy: Free
Original: Free
Green: 12

Preparation time 15 minutes
Cooking time about 2½ hours

low calorie cooking spray
600g/1lb 6oz boneless lamb shoulder, cut into large bite-sized pieces
2 large onions, peeled, halved and thickly sliced
3 garlic cloves, peeled and crushed
2 tsp finely grated root ginger
2 sticks of cassia bark or cinnamon
2 tsp chilli powder
2 tsp paprika
1 tsp crushed cardamom seeds
4 tbsp medium curry powder
400g can chopped tomatoes
1 tsp artificial sweetener
600ml/1 pint lamb stock
2 large carrots, peeled and cut into bite-sized pieces
300g/11oz swede, peeled and cut into bite-sized pieces
salt and freshly ground black pepper

TO SERVE
chopped coriander
whisked fat free natural yogurt

Spray a large, heavy-based flameproof casserole dish with low calorie cooking spray and place over a medium heat. Cook the lamb pieces in batches for 3–4 minutes until browned. Remove with a slotted spoon and set aside.

Spray the casserole dish again and add the onions. Cook over a medium heat for 10–12 minutes, stirring often, until soft and lightly browned.

Add the garlic, ginger, cassia bark or cinnamon, chilli powder, paprika and cardamom. Stir-fry for 1–2 minutes to release the aroma of the spices then add the curry powder and lamb. Stir-fry for 2–3 minutes then stir in the tomatoes, sweetener, stock, carrots and swede. Season well and bring to the boil.

Reduce the heat to very low and cover tightly. Simmer gently for 2 hours or until the lamb is meltingly tender. Remove from the heat, garnish with coriander, drizzle with yogurt and serve.

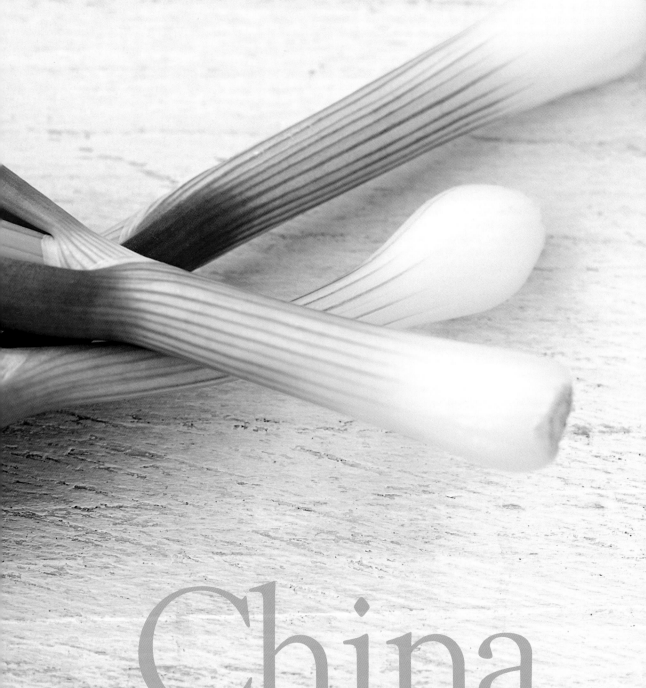

China

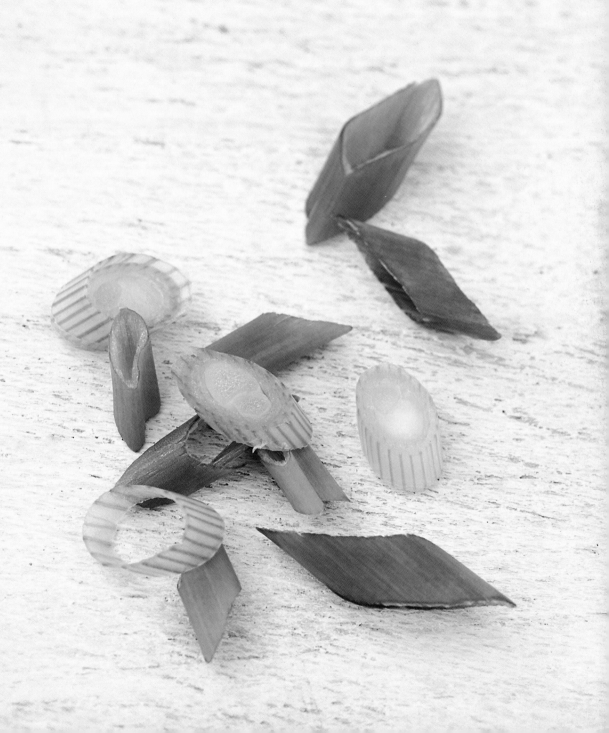

Spicy chicken noodle salad

Here is a delicious oriental salad made with succulent stir-fried chicken. Served warm or at room temperature, it makes a wonderful light lunch.

SERVES 4

EASY ✳

Syns per serving
Extra Easy: Free
Green: 4½
Original: 5½

Preparation time 10 minutes plus marinating
Cooking time 10 minutes

350g/12oz skinless chicken breast fillets, cut into thin strips
juice of 1 lemon or lime
½ tsp ground coriander
a pinch of Chinese five-spice powder
1 garlic clove, peeled and crushed
110g/4oz dried egg noodles
low calorie cooking spray
110g/4oz mangetout
1 red pepper, deseeded and thinly sliced
1 red chilli, deseeded and finely chopped
2.5cm/1in piece root ginger, peeled and chopped
2 tbsp soy sauce
salt and freshly ground black pepper

TO SERVE
torn coriander leaves

Put the chicken strips in a bowl with the lemon or lime juice, ground coriander, five-spice powder and garlic. Stir well to coat the chicken and set aside for 5 minutes to marinate.

Cook the noodles according to the packet instructions, until cooked and tender. Drain well.

Meanwhile, spray a wok or deep non-stick frying pan with low calorie cooking spray and place over a medium heat. Stir-fry the chicken strips, mangetout, pepper, chilli and ginger for 3–4 minutes, until the chicken is cooked and crisp.

Stir in the soy sauce and drained egg noodles. Toss well together and season. Cool a little before serving and garnish with coriander.

Spicy Szechuan noodles

Like most Szechuan food from western China, these noodles are served in a spicy sauce, flavoured with ginger and hot chillies. If you prefer a milder degree of heat, then only use one chilli.

SERVES 4

EASY ❊

Syns per serving
Extra Easy: ½
Green: 4
Original: 12

Preparation time 15 minutes
Cooking time 25 minutes

225g/8oz dried egg noodles
225g/8oz extra lean minced pork
2 tbsp soy sauce
1 tbsp sherry
low calorie cooking spray
2 garlic cloves, peeled and crushed
1 tbsp finely chopped root ginger
2 chillies, deseeded and finely chopped
4 spring onions, trimmed and sliced diagonally
½ red pepper, deseeded and sliced
8 baby sweetcorn
110g/4oz baby asparagus
1 tbsp miso (fermented soya bean paste)
150ml/¼ pint chicken stock
salt and freshly ground black pepper

TO SERVE
chopped chives

Cook the noodles according to the packet instructions, until tender. Drain and keep warm.

In a bowl mix the pork with the soy sauce and sherry. Place a wok or deep non-stick frying pan over a high heat and dry-fry the pork until it turns brown and is cooked through. Drain off any fat, transfer to a bowl and keep warm.

Wipe the wok or pan clean with kitchen paper. Spray with low calorie cooking spray and place over a medium heat. Add the garlic, ginger, chillies, spring onions, pepper, sweetcorn and asparagus. Stir-fry for 2 minutes, then stir in the miso. Cook for 1 minute, add the chicken stock and bring to the boil.

Reduce the heat a little and let the sauce simmer gently for about 5 minutes, until it reduces and thickens. Then add the pork and cook gently for another 2–3 minutes. Season, then mix the cooked noodles into the sauce.

Garnish the noodles with chopped chives and serve immediately.

Quick and easy stir-fried noodles

Syns per serving
Extra Easy: Free
Green: Free
Original: 11

Preparation time 10 minutes
Cooking time 8 minutes

225g/8oz dried egg noodles
low calorie cooking spray
2 baby aubergines, quartered
1 red pepper, deseeded
and thinly sliced
1 yellow pepper, deseeded
and thinly sliced
1 red chilli, deseeded
and finely chopped
4 spring onions, trimmed and sliced
110g/4oz baby sweetcorn
110g/4oz baby asparagus
4 tbsp soy sauce
25g/1oz basil or coriander, chopped

You can use virtually any vegetables with the cooked egg noodles in this classic Chinese dish.

Cook the noodles according to the packet instructions, until tender. Drain and keep warm.

Spray a wok or deep non-stick frying pan with low calorie cooking spray and place over a medium heat. When the wok or pan is hot, add the aubergines and stir-fry for 2–3 minutes, until they soften. Spray with a little low calorie cooking spray if necessary.

Add the peppers, chilli, spring onions, sweetcorn and asparagus, and continue stir-frying for about 3 minutes, until the sweetcorn and asparagus are just tender and have lost a little of their bite.

Add the noodles and soy sauce and gently toss with the vegetables. Cook for 1–2 minutes, until the noodles are heated through and everything is lightly coated with soy sauce.

Stir in the basil or coriander, remove from the heat and serve immediately.

Egg-fried rice

SERVES 4

EASY ❄ (only if prawns are fresh)

Syns per serving
Extra Easy: Free
Green: 4
Original: 6½

Preparation time 10 minutes
Cooking time 12–15 minutes

3 eggs
a pinch of salt
low calorie cooking spray
110g/4oz cooked and peeled prawns
110g/4oz cooked and
skinned chicken, diced
50g/2oz cooked peas
4 spring onions, trimmed and chopped
2 tbsp soy sauce
350g/12oz cold boiled rice
salt and freshly ground black pepper

This is a good way of using up leftover cold cooked rice or, of course, you can boil the rice especially for this dish. Serve with really fresh steamed vegetables dressed with a little soy sauce.

Beat the eggs and salt in a bowl. Heat a wok or deep non-stick frying pan and add the eggs. Stir over a gentle heat until the eggs have scrambled and set. Remove the eggs and set aside.

Spray the pan with low calorie cooking spray and place over a medium–high heat. Add the prawns, chicken, peas and spring onions. Stir-fry for 1 minute then stir in the soy sauce.

Continue stir-frying for a further 2 minutes, then add the rice and scrambled eggs. Stir constantly over a gentle heat until the rice is heated through. Season and serve immediately.

Steamed Chinese vegetables with smoked tofu

SERVES 4

EASY Ⓥ ⊛

Syns per serving
Extra Easy: ½
Original: ½
Green: ½

Preparation time 10 minutes plus marinating
Cooking time about 10 minutes

1 tbsp rice wine vinegar
4 tbsp soy sauce
1 large carrot, peeled and cut into matchsticks
200g/7oz broccoli florets
4 baby pak choi, halved
8 thin asparagus spears
10 shiitake mushrooms, halved
100g/3½oz smoked tofu, cut into bite-sized cubes
1 tsp sesame oil

Smoked tofu is available in most supermarkets and Asian greengrocers. If you can't find it, you can use firm, unsmoked tofu in its place.

Place the rice wine vinegar and soy sauce in a heatproof shallow bowl that will fit inside a steamer basket. Add the carrot and broccoli and marinate for about 10 minutes.

Bring a pan of water to the boil, fit the steamer basket, place the bowl inside, cover and steam the vegetables for 4–5 minutes.

Add the pak choi, asparagus and mushrooms, stirring to mix, cover and continue steaming for another 3 minutes.

Add the tofu, and continue steaming for 3–4 minutes until the vegetables are just softened. Remove the bowl from the steamer, toss gently with the sesame oil and serve immediately.

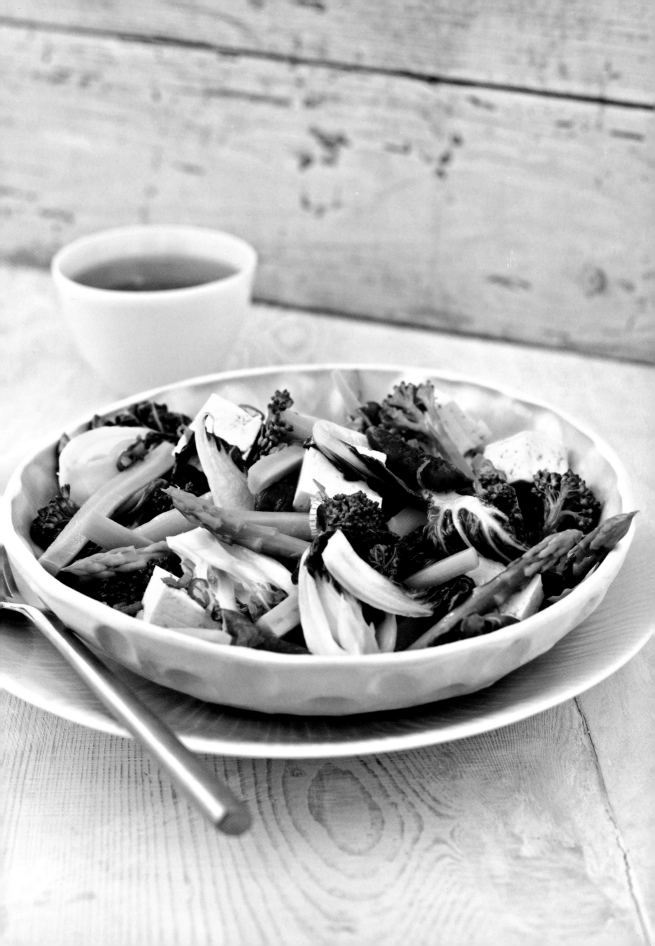

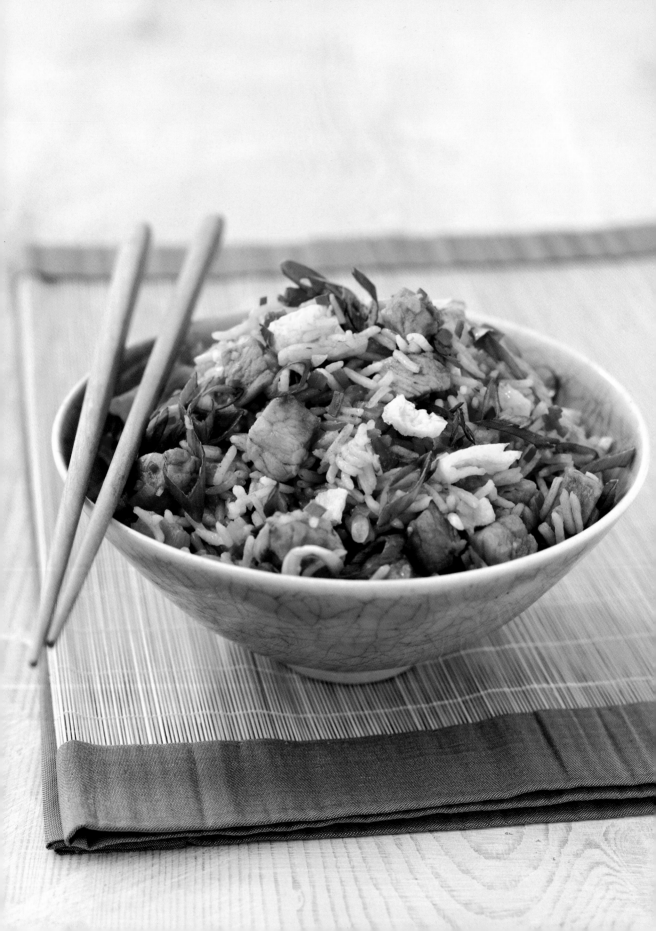

Special fried rice

SERVES 4

REALLY EASY ❋

Syns per serving
Extra Easy: Free
Green: 2½
Original: 8

Preparation time 10 minutes
Cooking time 12 minutes

low calorie cooking spray
1 garlic clove, peeled and crushed
3 tbsp soy sauce
150g/5oz lean pork fillet, diced
3 eggs
1 tbsp tomato purée
1 onion, peeled and finely chopped
450g/1lb cooked rice
4 spring onions, trimmed and chopped

TO SERVE
spring onion, sliced
2 tbsp chopped coriander
1 red chilli, deseeded and finely
chopped

Everybody who has eaten in a Chinese restaurant or enjoyed a Chinese takeaway is familiar with this recipe, but the rice is usually fried in oil and the finished dish is high in Syns. Here is a healthier version of an old favourite.

Spray a wok or deep non-stick frying pan with low calorie cooking spray and place over a medium heat. Add the garlic and cook for about 1 minute, until golden. Add 1 teaspoon of the soy sauce together with the pork and stir-fry for about 5 minutes until the pork is cooked through.

Break the eggs into the wok or pan and cook for about 2 minutes, stirring vigorously. Add the tomato purée, onion and the remaining soy sauce. Stir-fry for 1 minute, then add the rice and spring onions and continue cooking for about 4 minutes, until the rice is heated through.

Transfer the rice to a serving dish and garnish with the spring onion, coriander and chilli. Serve immediately.

Steamed sea bass with spring onion and ginger

SERVES 4

EASY ✻ (only if fish is fresh)

Syns per serving
Extra Easy: Free
Original: Free
Green: 9

Preparation time 20 minutes
Cooking time under 20 minutes

8 spring onions, trimmed and finely shredded
25g/1oz root ginger, peeled and cut into thin matchsticks
1 red chilli, deseeded and cut into fine strips
4 tbsp light soy sauce
2 tbsp rice wine vinegar
4 x 200g/7oz skinless sea bass fillets
4 banana leaf squares

The delicate flesh of the sea bass in this classic Chinese steamed fish dish is aromatically flavoured with ginger, spring onion, red chilli, soy sauce and rice wine vinegar.

Place the spring onions, ginger and chilli in a bowl and pour over the soy sauce and vinegar.

Place the sea bass fillets, skinned sides up, on a board and make six small cuts into each fillet.

Place a banana leaf or piece of baking parchment in the bottom of a steamer basket and place a sea bass fillet on top. Spoon a quarter of the spring onion mixture over the fillet. Repeat with the remaining banana leaves and fillets. (If you have a large steamer you should be able to fit two leaves in the basket.)

Place the lid on the steamer and set over a saucepan of boiling water. Steam for 8–10 minutes, or until just cooked through. Keep warm and repeat with the remaining leaves and fillets, then serve immediately.

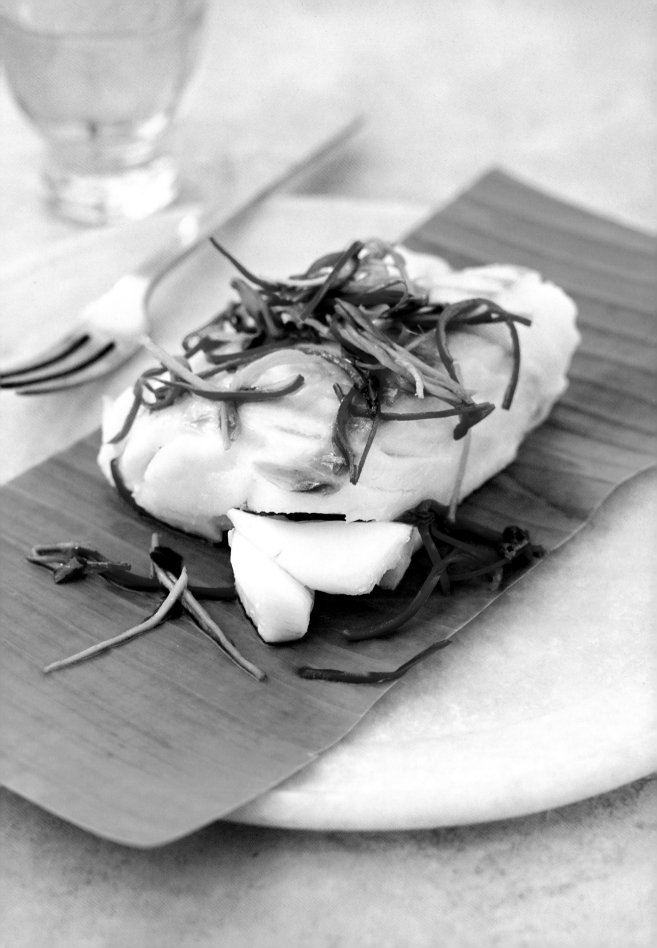

Sweet and sour prawns

SERVES 4

EASY ✻ (only if prawns are fresh)

Syns per serving
Extra Easy: 3
Original: 3
Green: 8½

Preparation time 20 minutes
Cooking time under 10 minutes

FOR THE SWEET AND SOUR SAUCE
1 tbsp white wine vinegar
2 tbsp soy sauce
1 tbsp tomato purée
1 tbsp sherry
6 tbsp unsweetened orange juice
1 tbsp brown sugar
1 tbsp cornflour

FOR THE PRAWNS
low calorie cooking spray
600g/1lb 6oz raw tiger prawns, peeled
1 garlic clove, peeled and crushed
4 spring onions, trimmed
and sliced diagonally
1 green pepper, deseeded and
cut into chunks
1 red pepper, deseeded and
cut into chunks
2 pineapple rings, canned
in juice and chopped
salt and freshly ground black pepper

Small bite-sized pieces of chicken or pork can be substituted for the prawns in this firm favourite – just cook for an extra 5–6 minutes or until the meat is cooked through.

To make the sweet and sour sauce, mix together all the sauce ingredients in a bowl until the cornflour is thoroughly blended.

Spray a wok or deep non-stick frying pan with low calorie cooking spray and place over a high heat. When it is very hot, add the prawns and stir-fry for 2–3 minutes until they turn pink. Add the garlic, spring onions and peppers and stir-fry for 2 minutes.

Add the pineapple then pour in the sweet and sour sauce. Keep stirring for 1 minute, turning the prawns and vegetables in the sauce until it thickens. Season and serve immediately.

Peking duck

One of the best-loved dishes in Chinese restaurants the world over, this is delicious food whatever the occasion.

Preheat the oven to 200°C/Gas 6. Spray a large non-stick frying pan with low calorie cooking spray and place over a high heat. Cook the duck breasts for 2–3 minutes on each side until browned. Transfer to a baking sheet and place in the oven. Roast for 20–25 minutes until cooked through. Remove from the oven and keep warm.

Meanwhile, make the pancakes. Sift the flour into a large bowl, mix the boiling water with half the oil and slowly stir into the flour. Knead to form a ball of warm dough.

Cut the dough in half and roll each half into a sausage, then cut each into eight equal pieces. Roll each one into a pancake approximately 15cm/6in across. Brush eight of the pancakes with the remaining oil and place an unoiled pancake on top of each one. Flatten each pair into a thin circle.

Heat the frying pan until it is very hot, then add one of the pancakes. Cook over a medium heat until air bubbles appear on the surface, then flip it over and cook the other side. Repeat with the remaining pancakes. Peel the two layers apart and keep the pancakes warm.

Shred the duck meat with a fork and place on a warmed serving dish. Arrange the spring onions and cucumber on a separate dish, and spoon the plum sauce into a bowl. To eat this dish, spread a little plum sauce on each pancake, top it with some duck, spring onions and cucumber, then roll it up.

Chicken chow mein

SERVES 4

EASY ✱

Probably the best-known noodle dish of all, chow mein can be stir-fried in a trice.

Syns per serving
Extra Easy: ½
Green: 3½
Original: 11½

Preparation time 15 minutes plus marinating
Cooking time 7–8 minutes

225g/8oz skinless chicken breast fillets, cut into thin strips
2 tbsp soy sauce
salt and freshly ground black pepper
225g/8oz dried egg noodles
low calorie cooking spray
1 onion, peeled and thinly sliced
2 garlic cloves, peeled and crushed
110g/4oz mangetout
110g/4oz beansprouts
4 spring onions, trimmed and shredded

TO SERVE
thin strips red chilli
2 tbsp chilli sauce (optional)

Place the chicken strips in a bowl with the soy sauce and seasoning. Stir the strips into the marinade and leave in a cool place for 15 minutes.

Cook the noodles according to the packet instructions until tender. Drain well.

Spray a wok or deep non-stick frying pan with low calorie cooking spray and place over a high heat until hot. Remove the chicken from the marinade (reserving any marinade) and add to the wok or pan. Stir-fry briskly for 2–3 minutes, until the chicken is cooked and golden. Remove and keep warm.

Add the onion, garlic, mangetout and beansprouts to the wok or pan and stir-fry for 2 minutes. Add the drained noodles and spring onions, return the chicken together with any leftover marinade and continue stir-frying for 1–2 minutes to heat through thoroughly. Garnish with strips of red chilli and serve immediately with the chilli sauce, if using.

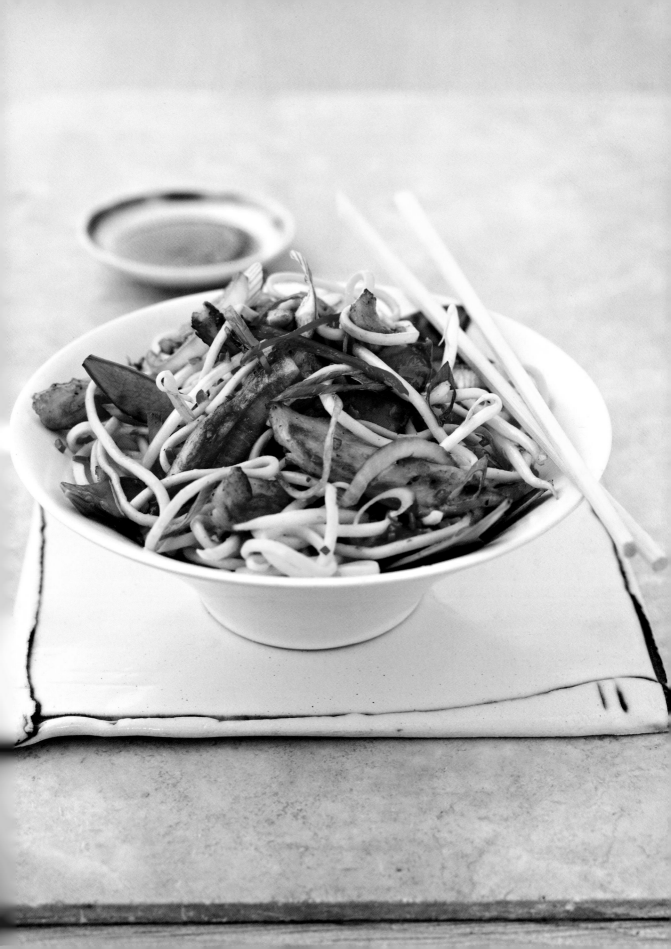

Cantonese pork in oyster sauce

Bottled oyster sauce is sold in most supermarkets and delicatessens. Surprisingly, although it's made from oysters it doesn't taste fishy and complements pork perfectly.

SERVES 4

WORTH THE EFFORT ❋

Syns per serving
Extra Easy: 1½
Original: 1½
Green: 9

Preparation time 15 minutes plus marinating
Cooking time 6–8 minutes

2 tbsp oyster sauce
1 tbsp soy sauce
1 tbsp sherry
2 tsp cornflour
500g/1lb 2oz lean pork fillets, cut into thin strips
low calorie cooking spray
2.5cm/1in piece root ginger, peeled and thinly sliced
4 spring onions, trimmed and sliced diagonally
2 carrots, peeled and cut into matchsticks
1 green pepper, deseeded and cut into chunks
1 tsp sugar
salt and freshly ground black pepper
2–3 tbsp chicken stock

Mix the oyster sauce, soy sauce, sherry and cornflour in a bowl. Add the strips of pork and turn them in the marinade until they are thoroughly coated, then cover and leave to marinate in a cool place for 30 minutes.

Spray a wok or deep non-stick frying pan with low calorie cooking spray and place over a medium–high heat. When hot, add the pork. Stir-fry for 2 minutes, or until sealed on the outside but still juicy inside. Remove and keep warm.

Add the ginger, spring onions, carrots and pepper to the wok or pan, and stir in the sugar. Stir-fry for 2 minutes, then add the pork, seasoning and stock. Stir-fry for 1 minute, turning the pork and vegetables in the sauce until warmed through and well coated. Serve immediately.

Pork in black bean sauce

SERVES 4

EASY ✳

Syns per serving
Extra Easy: 1
Original: 1
Green: 6

Preparation time 15 minutes plus
marinating
Cooking time 15 minutes

350g/12oz lean pork fillet
2 tbsp soy sauce
1 tbsp sherry
1 tsp cornflour
1 tsp grated root ginger
low calorie cooking spray
1 garlic clove, peeled and crushed
4 spring onions, trimmed
and sliced diagonally
1 green pepper, deseeded
and thinly sliced
2 tbsp black bean sauce
4 tbsp chicken stock

You can buy jars of black bean sauce, the essential ingredient in this recipe, in most supermarkets. This dish is usually made with spare ribs, but we have substituted pork fillet, which is much leaner.

Cut the pork into thin strips and place in a bowl with the soy sauce, sherry, cornflour and ginger. Mix together well, then cover and leave to marinate in a cool place for 30 minutes.

Spray a wok or deep non-stick frying pan with low calorie cooking spray and place over a high heat. When hot, add the pork and stir-fry for about 6 minutes, until it is cooked and golden. Remove, drain on kitchen paper and keep warm.

Add the garlic, spring onions and pepper to the wok and stir well. Stir-fry for 1 minute over a high heat, then add the black bean sauce and stock. Stir well and return the cooked pork to the mixture.

Reduce the heat to medium, cover and cook for 5 minutes, until the liquid has reduced and the pork and vegetables are coated with sauce. Serve immediately.

Szechuan beef

SERVES 4

EASY ⊛

Syns per serving
Extra Easy: ½
Original: ½
Green: 6

Preparation time 15 minutes plus marinating
Cooking time 8 minutes

1 tbsp soy sauce
2 tsp rice wine vinegar or white wine vinegar
½ tsp salt
1 tsp cornflour
2.5cm/1in piece root ginger, peeled and sliced
350g/12oz lean fillet, rump or sirloin steak, cut into strips
low calorie cooking spray
2 garlic cloves, peeled and crushed
1 red chilli, deseeded and thinly sliced
a good pinch of Chinese five-spice powder
1 red pepper, deseeded and cut into chunks
1 yellow pepper, deseeded and cut into chunks
1 tsp chilli sauce (optional)
freshly ground black pepper

TO SERVE
1 small red chilli, deseeded and cut into thin strips
1 spring onion, trimmed and finely sliced

This savoury dish is definitely for those of you who like spicy food. Szechuan is a province of western China and its food is characteristically piquant, with an emphasis on fiery chillies.

In a bowl, mix together the soy sauce, vinegar, salt, cornflour, ginger and 1 tablespoon of water. Add the strips of steak and turn them in the marinade. Cover and leave to marinate in the fridge or a cool place for 30 minutes.

Spray a wok or deep non-stick frying pan with low calorie cooking spray, place over a medium–high heat, and add the garlic, chilli and five-spice powder. Cook for 1 minute, then add the marinated steak strips. Stir-fry for a further 2–3 minutes, until the strips are brown outside but slightly pink and juicy inside. Remove and keep warm.

Add the peppers and stir-fry for 2 minutes, then return the steak and any remaining marinade to the wok or pan, together with the chilli sauce, if using. Stir-fry briskly over a medium heat for 1 minute. Season with plenty of black pepper.

Scatter the red chilli and spring onion over the top and serve immediately.

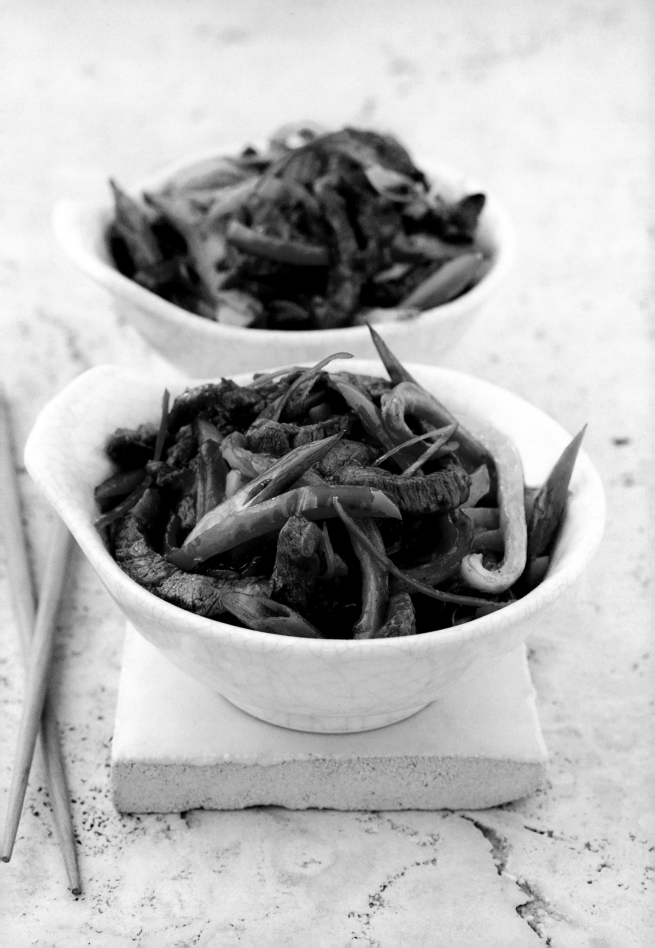

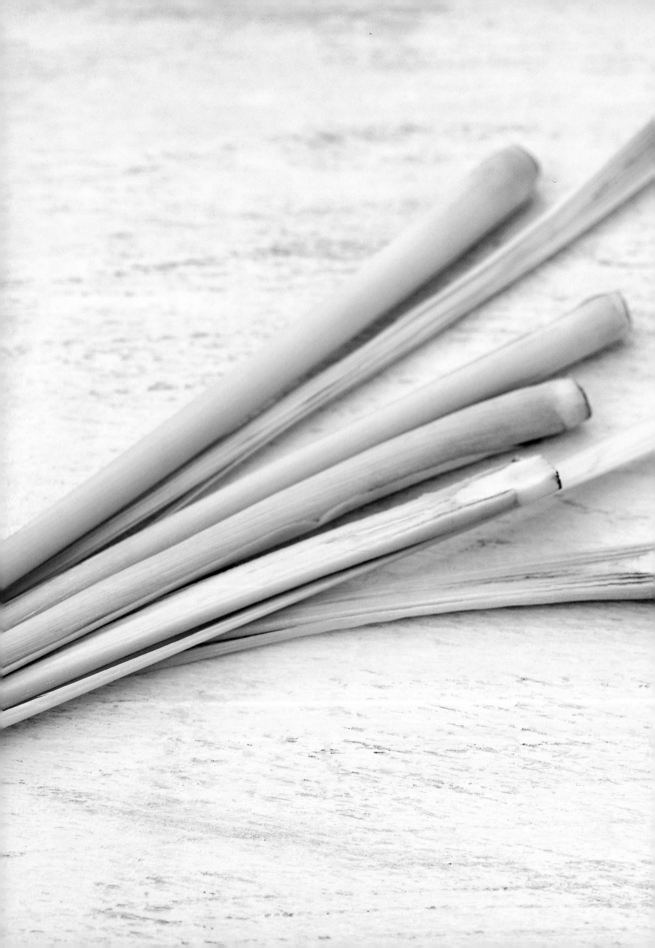

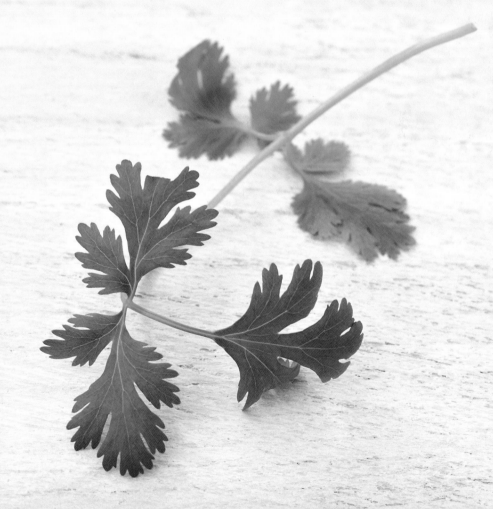

Thailand

Vegetable pad thai

Classic pad thai uses flat rice noodles, which are widely available from most supermarkets or Asian greengrocers. You could, however, use any type of cooked noodles for this dish.

SERVES 4

EASY (V) (✳)

Syns per serving
Extra Easy: ½
Green: ½
Original: 13

Preparation time 20 minutes
Cooking time under 10 minutes

250g pack medium rice noodles
2 tsp tamarind paste
3 tbsp nam pla (fish sauce)
2 tbsp dark soy sauce
1 tbsp sweet chilli sauce
¼ tsp artificial sweetener
2 garlic cloves, peeled and chopped
6 spring onions, trimmed and cut into 2cm/¾in slices
200g/7oz baby sweetcorn, cut into 2cm/¾in diagonal slices
1 large carrot, peeled and cut into thin matchsticks
1 red pepper, deseeded and cut into thin strips
100g/3½oz mangetout, trimmed and cut in half lengthways
1 egg
50g/2oz bean sprouts

TO SERVE
chopped coriander
lime halves

Prepare the noodles according to the packet instructions, drain well and keep warm.

Mix together the tamarind paste, nam pla, soy sauce, sweet chilli sauce and sweetener in a small bowl and set aside.

Spray a wok or deep non-stick frying pan with low calorie cooking spray and place over a high heat. When it is very hot add the garlic and spring onions and stir-fry for 30 seconds. Then add the sweetcorn, carrot, pepper and mangetout and stir-fry for 2–3 minutes.

Push the vegetables to the sides of the wok or pan. Crack the egg into the centre and keep stirring it for 30 seconds or so, until it begins to set and resembles a broken-up omelette.

Add the beansprouts, followed by the drained noodles, then pour the nam pla mixture over the top. Toss everything together and heat through.

Spoon on to plates, garnish with chopped coriander and serve with lime halves to squeeze over.

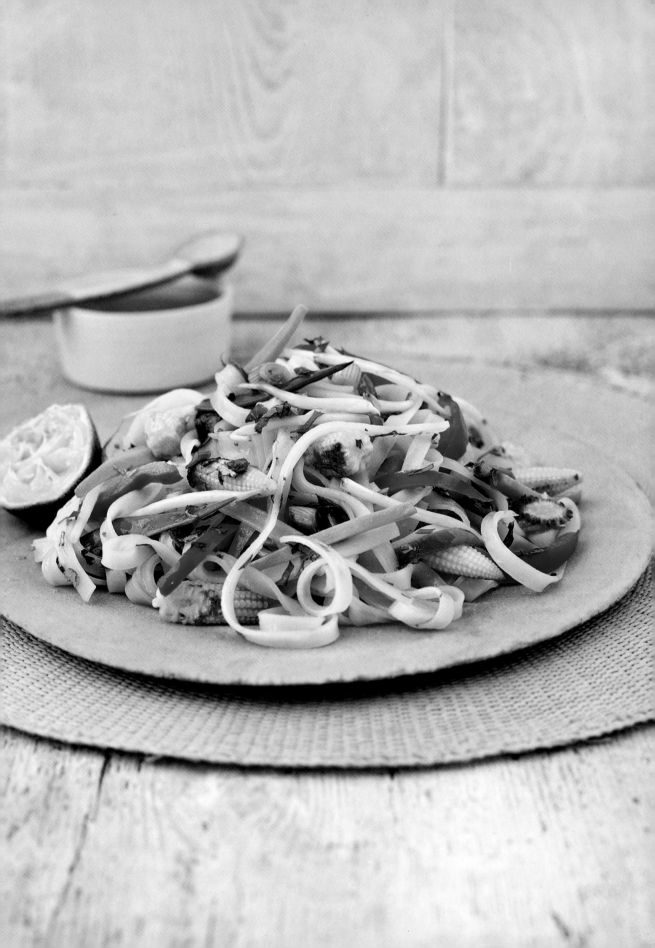

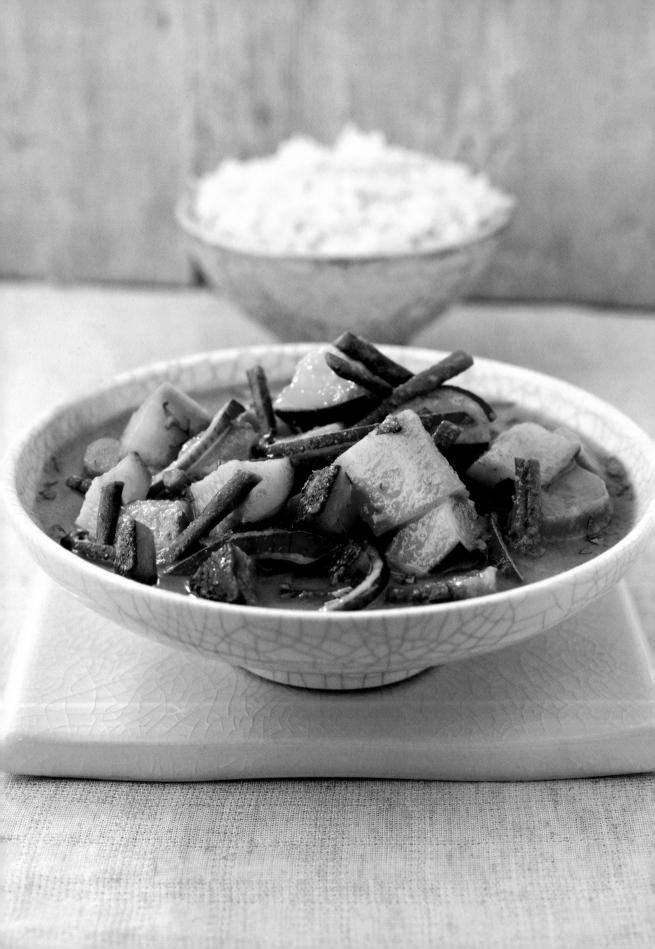

Thai fragrant vegetable curry

SERVES 4

WORTH THE EFFORT (V)(✱)

Syns per serving
Extra Easy: 1
Green: 1
Original: 11½

Preparation time 15 minutes
Cooking time 20 minutes

FOR THE CURRY PASTE
2 garlic cloves, peeled and crushed
1 lemongrass stalk, chopped
1 Thai red chilli, deseeded and chopped
a small bunch of coriander
1 spring onion, trimmed and chopped
1 tsp crushed coriander seeds

FOR THE THAI FRAGRANT CURRY
low calorie cooking spray
1 red onion, peeled and thinly sliced
2 courgettes, cut into chunks
1 aubergine, cubed
2 large carrots, peeled and cut into chunks
110g/4oz thin green beans
90ml/3fl oz canned light coconut milk
200ml/7fl oz vegetable stock
juice of 1 lime
salt and freshly ground black pepper
225g/8oz dried long-grain rice

TO SERVE
chopped coriander

This aromatic and creamy vegetable curry is great for hassle-free entertaining as it can be made in advance and just heated through before serving.

To make the curry paste, blend all the ingredients with an electric hand-held blender or pound in a pestle and mortar until they are smooth.

Spray a large saucepan with low calorie cooking spray and place over a medium heat. Add the onion, courgettes, aubergine and carrots and cook, stirring, for about 5 minutes until golden.

Stir in the curry paste and cook for 1 minute before adding the beans, coconut milk and stock. Simmer gently for 15 minutes, then stir in the lime juice, and season.

Meanwhile, cook the rice according to the packet instructions and drain thoroughly. Scatter chopped coriander over the vegetables and serve the curry with the rice.

Green curry vegetable fried rice

SERVES 4

EASY (V)(❄)

Syns per serving
Extra Easy: 1
Green: 1
Original: 9

Preparation time 15–20 minutes
Cooking time under 10 minutes

low calorie cooking spray
3 garlic cloves, peeled and finely sliced
1 tsp finely chopped root ginger
4 spring onions, trimmed
and finely sliced
1 tsp ready-made green curry paste
(or see recipe page 184)
300g/11oz cold boiled long-grain rice
4 tbsp canned light coconut milk
100g/3½oz tenderstem broccoli,
cut into bite-sized pieces and blanched
100g/3½oz carrots, cut into thin
matchsticks and blanched
1 red pepper, deseeded and cut
into very thin strips
200g/7oz canned sweetcorn kernels,
drained and rinsed
100g/3½oz mangetout,
halved lengthways
2 tbsp chopped coriander
1 tbsp light soy sauce

If you don't want to use shop-bought green curry paste in this dish, you can make your own Syn-Free version using the recipe in Thai Chicken Curry (page 184).

Spray a wok or deep non-stick frying pan with low calorie cooking spray and place over a medium heat. When hot, add the garlic, ginger, spring onions and green curry paste. Stir-fry for 30 seconds, then add the rice, coconut milk, vegetables and coriander.

Stir-fry for 3–4 minutes then sprinkle with the soy sauce. Remove from the heat and serve immediately.

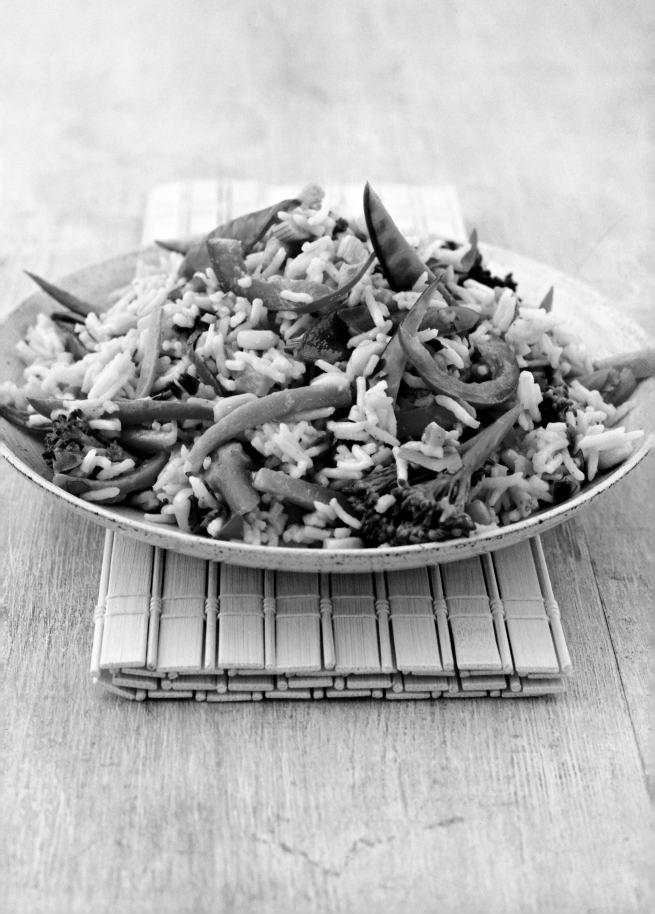

Spicy prawn soup

SERVES 6

EASY (❋) (only if prawns are fresh)

Syns per serving
Extra Easy: Free
Original: Free
Green: 3

Preparation time 10 minutes
Cooking time 25–30 minutes

1 tbsp finely chopped lemongrass
4 kaffir lime leaves (optional)
1 tbsp nam pla (fish sauce)
450g/1lb raw tiger prawns, peeled
juice of 2 limes
4 spring onions, trimmed
and thinly sliced
1 Thai red bird's eye chilli, deseeded
and cut into thin strips
4 tbsp chopped coriander
salt and freshly ground black pepper

TO SERVE
a few coriander sprigs

This fragrant soup is a popular dish in Thailand. Nowadays, there are no problems getting authentic Thai ingredients as most supermarkets sell kaffir lime leaves, nam pla (fish sauce), lemongrass and the small Thai red bird's eye chillies.

Bring 2 litres/3½ pints of water to the boil in a large saucepan. Add the lemongrass, and lime leaves, if using, and simmer for 10 minutes. Add the nam pla and continue simmering gently for 5 minutes.

Add the prawns and lime juice and cook over a very low heat for about 5 minutes, or until the prawns turn pink.

Add the spring onions, chilli and coriander to the pan and cook for 2 minutes before checking the seasoning (the nam pla is quite salty so you may not need to add any salt).

Garnish with coriander sprigs and serve immediately.

Thai crabcakes

SERVES 4

EASY ❄

Syns per serving
Extra Easy: 2
Original: 2
Green: 5

Preparation time 10 minutes plus
chilling
Cooking time 1 hour

These spicy crabcakes are delicious simply served with a crisp salad and a tangy tomato salsa.

FOR THE TOMATO SALSA
2 garlic cloves, unpeeled
low calorie cooking spray
3 tomatoes, skinned, deseeded and chopped
½ red onion, peeled and finely chopped
1 small red pepper, roasted, skinned, deseeded and chopped
1 Thai red bird's eye chilli, deseeded and finely chopped
2 tbsp chopped coriander
juice of ½ lime

FOR THE CRABCAKES
350g/12oz canned crab meat, drained
a small bunch of coriander, chopped
1 red chilli, deseeded and finely chopped
4 spring onions, trimmed and chopped
1 tsp nam pla (fish sauce)
1 stalk lemongrass, finely chopped
1 egg, beaten
1 tbsp reduced calorie mayonnaise
25g/1oz dried breadcrumbs

Preheat the oven to 190°C/Gas 5. Place the garlic on a piece of foil, spray with low calorie cooking spray and season well. Seal the foil and roast in the oven for 50 minutes. Peel the garlic cloves, place in a bowl and mash with a fork. Mix with the remaining salsa ingredients and set aside.

Meanwhile, prepare the crabcakes. Put the crab meat in a bowl and mix in the coriander, chilli, spring onions, nam pla and lemongrass. Bind the mixture with the egg, mayonnaise and breadcrumbs.

Chill the mixture in the fridge for 10–15 minutes, then divide into eight equal portions. Shape each one into a round flat cake and spray lightly with low calorie cooking spray.

Preheat the grill to hot and cook the crabcakes for 4–5 minutes on each side, until golden brown.

Serve immediately with the salsa.

Lemongrass prawn skewers

SERVES 4

EASY

Syns per serving
Extra Easy: 1
Original: 1
Green: 6½

Preparation time 20 minutes
Cooking time under 10 minutes

600g/1lb 6oz minced raw tiger prawns
2 tbsp chopped lemongrass
10 tbsp finely chopped coriander
5 tbsp finely chopped mint
2 tbsp soy sauce
1 tbsp grated root ginger
2–3 garlic cloves, peeled and crushed
1 red chilli, deseeded and
finely chopped
1 tbsp nam pla (fish sauce)
12 lemongrass stalks
low calorie cooking spray
salt and freshly ground black pepper

TO SERVE
2 tbsp sweet chilli sauce

Here, minced prawns flavoured with aromatic Thai herbs and spices are moulded around fresh lemongrass stalks to impart a fragrant flavour to the kebabs.

In a large bowl, combine the minced prawns with the chopped lemongrass, chopped herbs, soy sauce, ginger, garlic, red chilli and nam pla.

Using wet hands, divide the mixture into 12 portions and press around a lemongrass stalk to form a sausage shape around it. Transfer the prawn skewers to a baking sheet.

Preheat the grill to medium–hot. Spray the skewers lightly with low calorie cooking spray and season. Cover the ends of the skewers with foil and place under the grill for about 7 minutes, turning once or twice, until the kebabs are browned and just cooked through. Transfer the skewers to a large serving plate, and serve with the sweet chilli sauce.

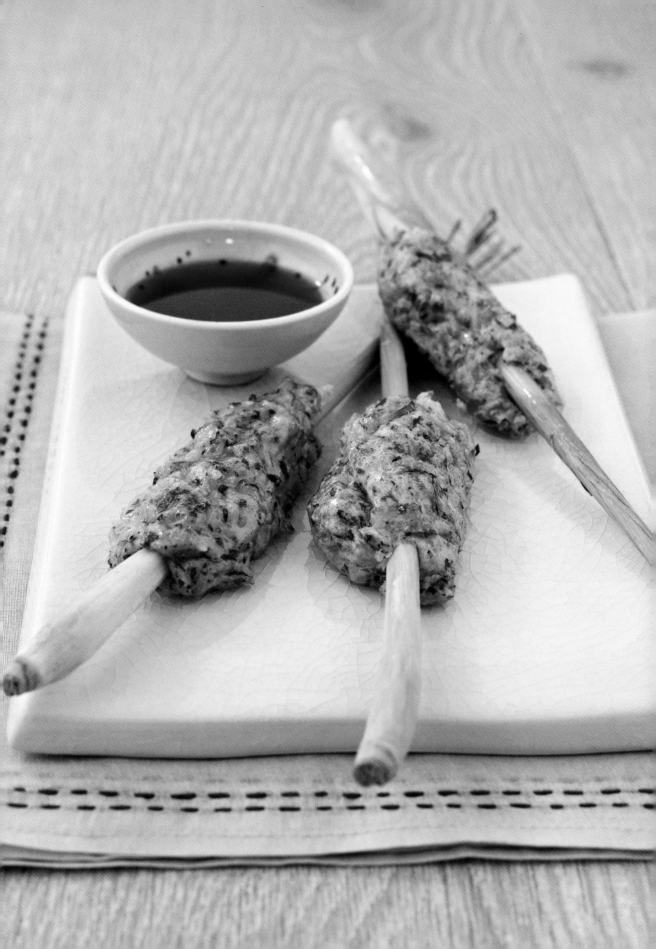

Thai chicken curry

SERVES 4

WORTH THE EFFORT ✳

Syns per serving
Extra Easy: 2½
Original: 2½
Green: 9

Preparation time 15 minutes
Cooking time 25 minutes

FOR THE GREEN CURRY PASTE
4 green chillies, deseeded and chopped
2.5cm/1in piece root ginger, peeled
and finely chopped
2 stalks lemongrass, finely chopped
2 garlic cloves, peeled and crushed
1 small onion, peeled and finely chopped
grated rind and juice of 1 lime
½ tsp coriander seeds, crushed
1 tsp ground cumin
½ tsp black peppercorns

FOR THE CHICKEN CURRY
low calorie cooking spray
450g/1lb skinless chicken breast fillets,
cut into large strips
2 tbsp green curry paste (see above)
150ml/¼ pint chicken stock
50g/2oz coconut cream
4 kaffir lime leaves
½ level tsp brown sugar
1 tbsp nam pla (fish sauce)

TO SERVE
2 red or green chillies, deseeded
and thinly sliced
freshly ground black pepper
torn basil leaves

If you haven't tried a Thai curry, now is the moment to discover this gastronomic pleasure. You can buy ready-made green curry paste, but this would add Syns to the recipe, so here's our very own Syn-Free version. If covered, it keeps in the fridge for up to a week.

To make the green curry paste, put all the ingredients in a bowl and blend until smooth.

To make the chicken curry, spray a large non-stick frying pan with low calorie cooking spray and place over a medium–high heat. Sauté the chicken strips for 2–3 minutes, then add the green curry paste. Cook for 1 minute, then add the stock and simmer for about 10 minutes, until the stock reduces.

Add the coconut cream, lime leaves, sugar and nam pla. Cook gently for 10 minutes, until the chicken is cooked.

Garnish the curry with the chilli slices, black pepper and torn basil leaves, and serve.

Fragrant stir-fried chicken with rice

SERVES 4

EASY ✳

Syns per serving
Extra Easy: ½
Original: 4
Green: 5

Preparation time 15 minutes
Cooking time 8–10 minutes

low calorie cooking spray
350g/12oz skinless chicken breast
fillets, cut into thin strips
1 lemongrass stalk, finely chopped
2.5cm/1in piece root ginger, peeled
and finely chopped
1–2 Thai red bird's eye chillies,
deseeded and finely chopped
1 red pepper, deseeded and
cut into thin strips
1 yellow pepper, deseeded and
cut into thin strips
1 tbsp medium/dry sherry
2 tbsp soy sauce

TO SERVE
a few coriander leaves,
roughly chopped
225g/8oz boiled Thai fragrant rice

It's worth keeping a few Thai ingredients in the fridge so that you can make this recipe when you need to rustle up a quick and easy meal. Most supermarkets sell little packs of lemongrass, Thai red bird's eye chillies and fresh coriander.

Spray a wok or deep non-stick frying pan with low calorie cooking spray and place over a high heat. When it is really hot, add the chicken strips and stir-fry for about 3 minutes, until the chicken is cooked. Remove the chicken and keep warm.

Add the lemongrass, ginger, chillies and peppers to the wok or pan and stir-fry for 2–3 minutes. Return the chicken to the wok or pan, together with the sherry and soy sauce.

Continue cooking for 2 minutes, until the liquid has reduced. Sprinkle with chopped coriander and serve the stir-fried chicken immediately with the Thai fragrant rice.

Spicy minced pork on lettuce leaves

Syns per serving
Extra Easy: ½
Original: ½
Green: 8½

Preparation time 20 minutes
Cooking time 12–15 minutes

2 tbsp finely chopped lemongrass
2 lime leaves, finely shredded
2 red chillies, deseeded and
finely chopped
3 garlic cloves, peeled and finely diced
2 tbsp finely diced root ginger
low calorie cooking spray
500g/1lb 2oz extra lean minced pork
1 tsp sweet chilli sauce
60ml/2fl oz nam pla (fish sauce)
6 spring onions, trimmed and
finely sliced
3 tbsp lime juice
a handful each of basil, coriander and
mint leaves, roughly chopped

TO SERVE
2 little gem lettuces, leaves separated
50g/2oz beansprouts
lime wedges

Known as 'larb' in Thai – a spicy meat salad flavoured with fish sauce – this mince mixture can be made with any lean minced meat of your choice.

Place the lemongrass, lime leaves, chillies, garlic and ginger into a food processor and blend until everything is very finely chopped.

Spray a wok or deep non-stick frying pan with low calorie cooking spray and place over a high heat. Add the lemongrass mixture and pork and stir-fry for 4–5 minutes, until the meat is browned all over, then add the sweet chilli sauce and nam pla.

Turn down the heat a little and allow the mixture to cook for 5–6 minutes, stirring often, then add the spring onions and cook for another minute.

Remove the wok or pan from the heat, pour the lime juice over the pork, add the herbs and toss. Serve the pork in the lettuce leaves and accompany with the beansprouts, and lime wedges to squeeze over.

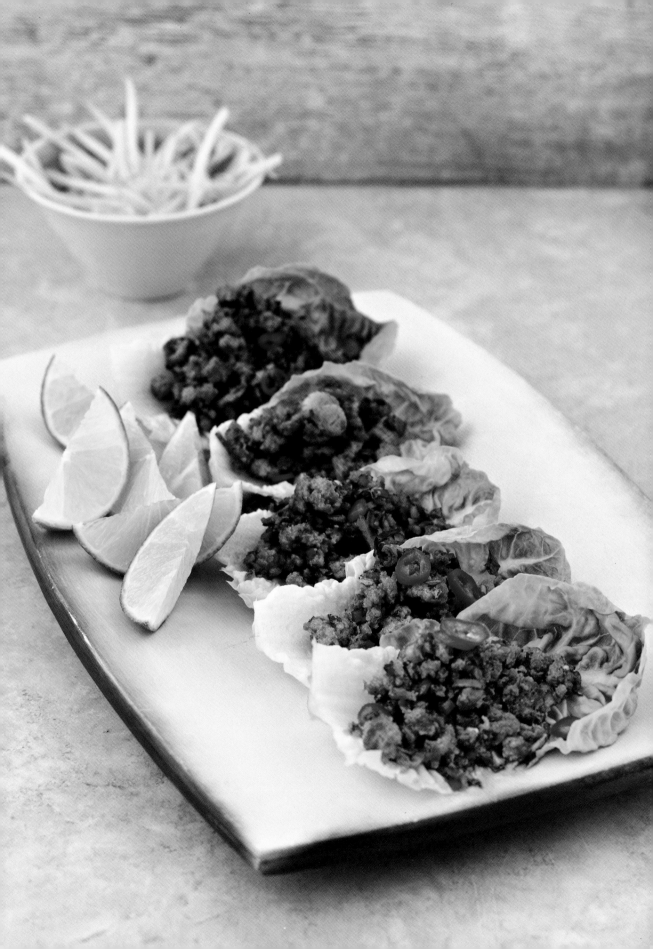

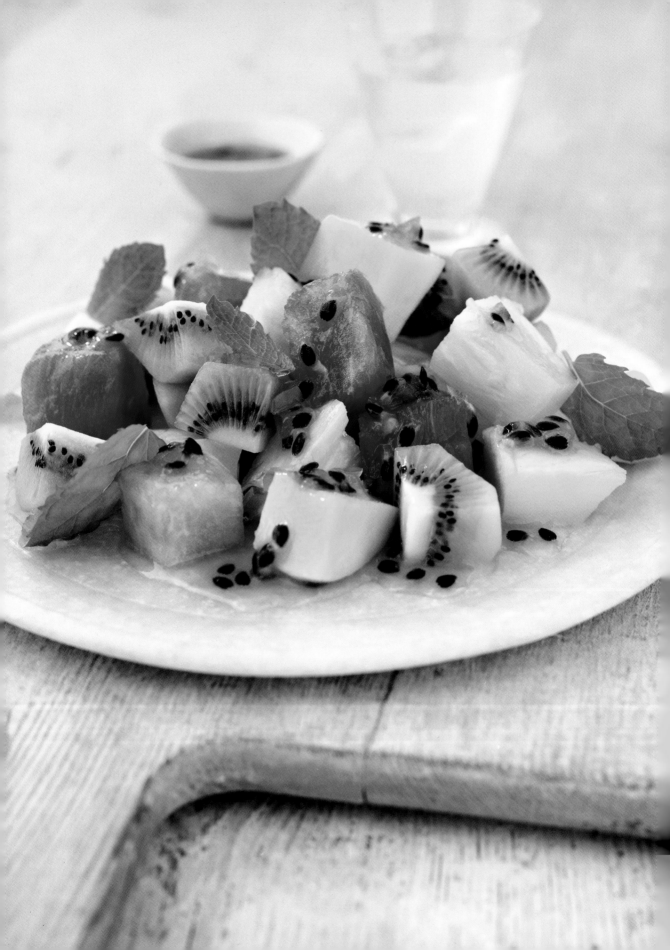

Tropical fruit salad with passion fruit and sweet ginger dressing

SERVES 4

EASY ⊛

Syns per serving
Extra Easy: 1½
Original: 1½
Green: 1½

Preparation time 25 minutes

4 kiwi fruit, peeled and cut into
1.5cm/½in pieces
1 papaya, peeled and cut into
1.5cm/½in pieces
2 mangoes, peeled, stoned and cut
into bite-sized cubes
¼ pineapple, cut into cubes
½ small watermelon, cut into cubes

FOR THE DRESSING
1 tbsp stem ginger, very finely diced
juice and pulp of 2 passion fruit
1 tbsp runny honey
¼ tsp ground ginger
artificial sweetener, to taste (optional)

TO SERVE
mint leaves

Refreshing, colourful and sweet tropical fruits are tossed together with a passion fruit and ginger dressing and can be served chilled or at room temperature.

Place all the fruit in a large serving bowl and toss to mix well.

To make the dressing, place the stem ginger, passion fruit pulp and juice, honey and ground ginger in a small saucepan with 200ml/7fl oz of water, and the sweetener, if using. Stir to mix well and bring to the boil. Remove from the heat and allow to cool for 5–6 minutes.

Drizzle the dressing over the fruit salad, garnish with mint leaves, and serve.

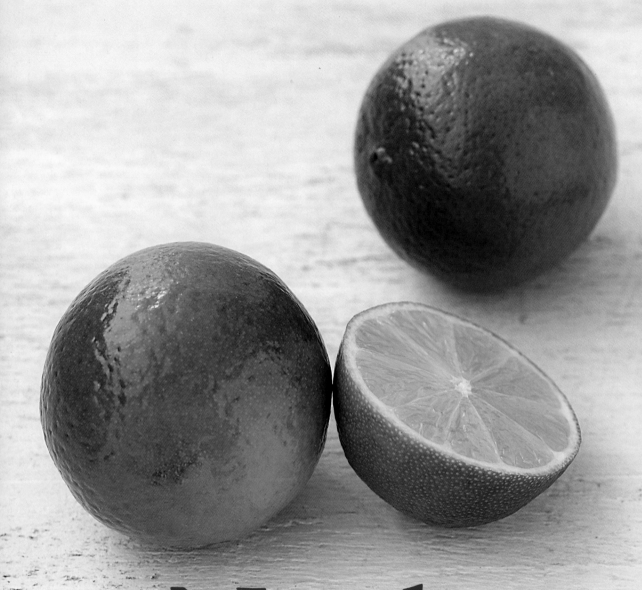

North America

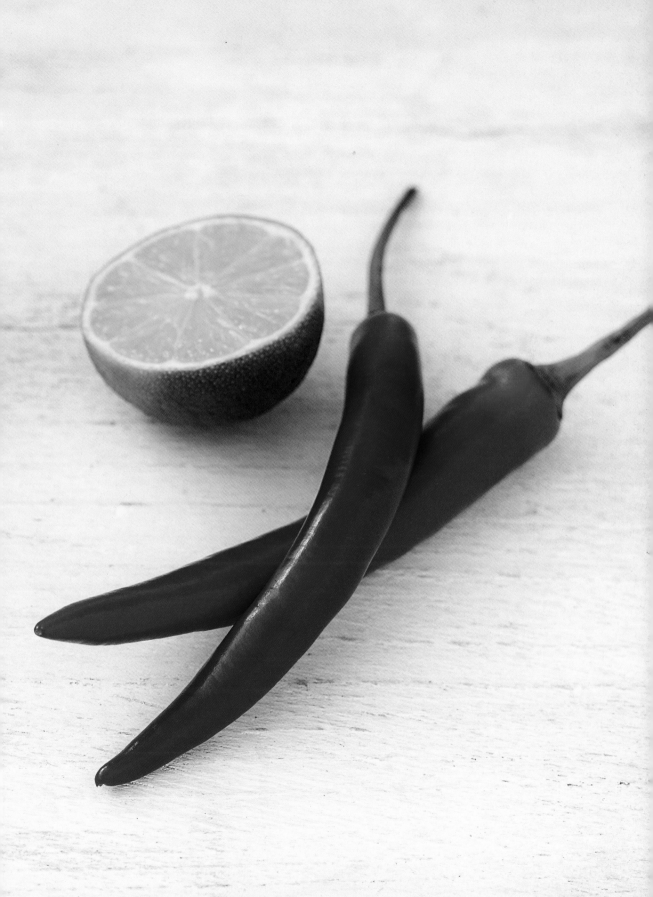

Manhattan clam chowder

Many recipes exist for this all-American dish, usually enriched with cream, but this version from New York's Manhattan is a healthier alternative, flavoured with tomatoes instead of cream.

SERVES 4

EASY ❋

Syns per serving
Extra Easy: Free
Original: 2
Green: 2

Preparation time 15 minutes
Cooking time 1¼ hours

2 large onions, peeled and chopped
2 leeks, trimmed and finely chopped
1 large red pepper, deseeded and chopped
900ml/1½ pints fish or vegetable stock
400g can chopped tomatoes
½ tsp dried thyme
225g/8oz potatoes, peeled and cubed
225g/8oz clams canned in brine, drained
salt and freshly ground black pepper
a dash of Tabasco sauce

TO SERVE
2 tbsp chopped flat-leaf parsley

Put the onions, leeks, pepper and one-third of the stock in a large heavy-based saucepan, cover and bring to the boil. Boil for 5–10 minutes, until the vegetables are beginning to soften, then uncover and simmer gently for 20–30 minutes, until the onions are tender, golden and syrupy.

Add the remaining stock and the tomatoes and thyme and simmer gently for 15 minutes. Then add the potatoes and clams. Season and simmer for a further 15 minutes, until the potatoes are cooked and tender but not mushy.

Check the seasoning, add the Tabasco sauce, sprinkle with the parsley and serve.

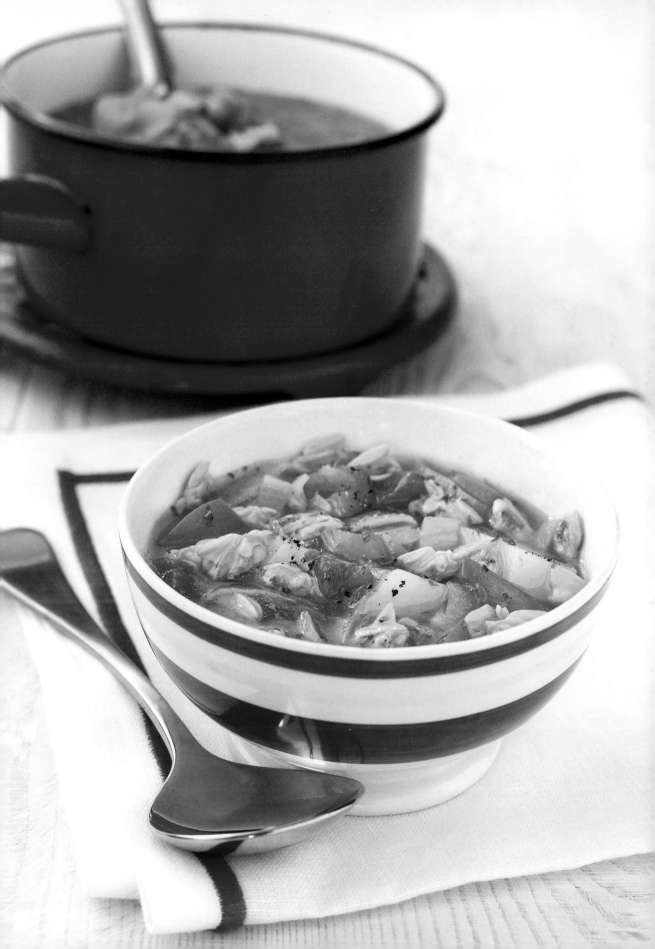

New England corn chowder

SERVES 4

REALLY EASY

This quick, easy and hearty soup makes a great warming autumnal or winter supper.

Syns per serving
Extra Easy: Free
Green: Free
Original: 10½

Preparation time 10 minutes
Cooking time 25–30 minutes

low calorie cooking spray
1 large onion, peeled and
finely chopped
1 large potato, peeled and
cut into 1cm/½in dice
1 garlic clove, peeled and crushed
800ml/28fl oz vegetable stock
400g/14oz canned creamed sweetcorn
400g/14oz canned sweetcorn kernels,
drained and rinsed
4 tbsp chopped parsley
salt and freshly ground black pepper

Spray a large non-stick frying pan with low calorie cooking spray and place over a medium heat. Add the onion, potato, garlic and stock and bring to the boil.

Add the creamed sweetcorn and sweetcorn kernels and return to the boil. Reduce the heat, cover and cook for 10–15 minutes.

Remove from the heat, stir in the parsley and season well. Ladle into warmed bowls and serve.

Mexican black bean soup

SERVES 4

WORTH THE EFFORT Ⓥ ❋

Syns per serving
Extra Easy: Free
Green: Free
Original: 17

Preparation time 20 minutes plus overnight soaking
Cooking time 2 hours

500g/1lb 2oz dried black beans
2 onions, peeled and roughly chopped
2 celery sticks, roughly chopped
2 large carrots, peeled and roughly chopped
3 garlic cloves, peeled and chopped
1 bouquet garni (parsley and thyme sprigs and 2 bay leaves)
2 x 400g cans chopped tomatoes
1 heaped tbsp cumin seeds
1 tbsp dried oregano
juice of 1 lime
salt and freshly ground black pepper

TO SERVE
6 spring onions, trimmed and thinly sliced
2 red chillies, deseeded and very finely chopped
a small bunch of coriander, roughly chopped
1–2 limes, cut into wedges

This robust and flavoursome soup makes for great entertaining as guests can help themselves to the toppings of their choice. Serve with steamed rice and salad for a main meal, if desired.

Soak the beans for four hours (or overnight) in a bowl of cold water, then drain in a colander.

Spray a large heavy-based saucepan with low calorie cooking spray and place over a medium heat. Add the onions, celery, carrots, garlic and bouquet garni, cover and leave to sweat on a low heat for 10–15 minutes, until the vegetables are juicy and tender.

Add the beans and enough water to cover the contents of the pan by about 8cm/3in. Don't add salt at this stage or the beans won't soften as they cook.

Bring to the boil and boil hard for 10 minutes, then reduce the heat and simmer gently, covered, for 50 minutes–1¼ hours, until the beans are very tender.

Add the tomatoes, cumin seeds, oregano, lime juice, and season well. Simmer for another 30 minutes, stirring occasionally with a wooden spoon and crushing some of the beans against the side of the pan (you can use an electric hand-held blender if you like a thicker soup). At the end of cooking, remove the bouquet garni.

Put the spring onions, chillies, coriander and lime wedges into bowls and arrange them on the table so that guests can select their favourite toppings. Ladle the hot soup into warmed bowls and serve.

Waldorf salad

SERVES 4

EASY (V)

Syns per serving
Extra Easy: 4
Original: 4
Green: 4

Preparation time 20–25 minutes

FOR THE DRESSING
10 tbsp extra light mayonnaise
2 tsp white wine vinegar
1 tsp Dijon mustard
a pinch of artificial sweetener
salt and freshly ground black pepper

FOR THE SALAD
1 medium celeriac
juice of 1 lemon
2 apples, cored
2 ripe pears, cored
4 celery sticks, finely sliced
2 little gem lettuces, leaves separated
25g/1oz chopped walnuts

This very easy, simple salad has a long, rich history. It was created in the 1890s at New York's Waldorf-Astoria Hotel by maître d' Oscar Tschirky. The original salad contained only mayonnaise, red apples and celery, but today it is usually made with walnuts, celeriac and other ingredients.

To make the dressing, place the mayonnaise, vinegar, mustard and sweetener in a bowl and blend to combine. Season to taste and set aside until needed.

For the salad, peel the celeriac and cut into manageable chunks. Using a mandolin, slice the celeriac pieces into thin strips. Place them immediately into a large bowl with some of the lemon juice and just enough water to cover. Prepare the apples and pears in exactly the same way.

Drain the celeriac, apples and pears and toss them in the dressing along with the celery. Season. Line a large serving bowl with the lettuce leaves and top with the salad. Scatter with the walnuts and serve.

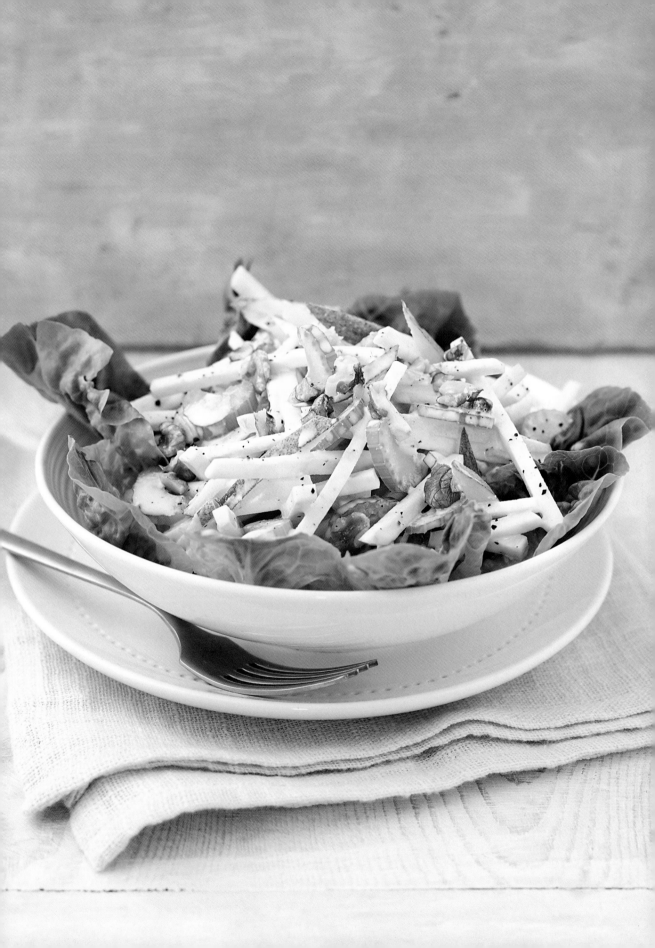

Caesar salad

SERVES 4

EASY

Syns per serving
Extra Easy: 4
Original: 4
Green: 5½

Preparation time 15 minutes
Cooking time 5–10 minutes

2 x 25g/1oz slices crusty white bread
2 garlic cloves, peeled and crushed
2 tsp olive oil
1 large cos lettuce, leaves separated
and torn if large
50g/2oz anchovy fillets canned in oil,
drained and chopped

FOR THE DRESSING
90ml/3fl oz fat free vinaigrette
2 egg yolks, beaten
1 tsp Dijon mustard
juice of 1 lemon
a dash of Worcestershire sauce
salt and freshly ground black pepper
3 tbsp grated Parmesan cheese

The renowned Caesar salad was created by Alex-Caesar Cardini in 1926 but is usually a no-go for anyone watching their weight as the dressing in particular is very high in calories. Now you can enjoy a special low-Syn version of the classic recipe.

Preheat the oven to 180°C/Gas 4. Cut the bread into small dice, place in a bowl with the garlic and olive oil and toss lightly. Place the croûtons on a baking sheet and cook in the oven for 5–10 minutes, until they are crisp and golden. Set aside to cool.

Put the lettuce leaves in a large bowl with the drained anchovies and add the cooled croûtons.

To make the dressing, blend together all the ingredients and pour over the lettuce, anchovies and croûtons. Toss gently and serve the salad immediately.

Macaroni cheese

Spring onions, cherry tomatoes and peas make a colourful and tasty addition to this family-friendly pasta dish.

SERVES 4

EASY (V) (❋)

Syns per serving
Extra Easy: 6
Green: 6
Original: 25

Preparation time 15 minutes
Cooking time about 25 minutes

400g/14oz dried macaroni
low calorie cooking spray
6 spring onions, trimmed and thinly sliced
2 garlic cloves, peeled and chopped
300g/11oz cherry tomatoes, halved
200g/7oz frozen peas
150ml/¼ pint vegetable stock

FOR THE TOPPING
500g/1lb 2oz fat free natural yogurt
1 tsp Dijon mustard
175g/6oz reduced fat Cheddar cheese, coarsely grated
2 eggs, lightly beaten
4 tbsp very finely chopped parsley
salt and freshly ground black pepper

TO SERVE
vegetables or a mixed salad

Cook the macaroni according to the packet instructions until just tender. Drain well.

Meanwhile, spray a large non-stick frying pan with low calorie cooking spray and place over a high heat. Add the spring onions, garlic, cherry tomatoes and peas and stir and cook for 2–3 minutes. Add the stock to the pan and cook for 6–8 minutes or until it has been absorbed.

Stir in the drained macaroni and toss to mix well. Transfer this mixture to a shallow ovenproof dish.

Preheat the oven to 220°C/Gas 7. Make the topping by mixing together all the ingredients in a bowl, seasoning well. Pour over the macaroni mixture. Place in the oven and cook for 15–20 minutes, or until lightly golden and bubbling. Remove and leave to stand for 5 minutes before serving. Accompany with vegetables or a mixed salad.

Mexican burritos

You'll love these spicy tortilla parcels filled with chickpeas in a tomato sauce. Serve them with vegetables or a crisp green salad.

SERVES 4

EASY Ⓥ ❄

Syns per serving
Extra Easy: 5½
Green: 5½
Original: 9

Preparation time 15 minutes
Cooking time 1¼ hours

FOR THE FILLING
1 onion, peeled and chopped
1 garlic clove, peeled and crushed
300ml/½ pint vegetable stock
1 red pepper, deseeded and chopped
1 red chilli, deseeded and chopped
225g/8oz tomatoes, skinned
and chopped
225g/8oz canned chickpeas, drained
and rinsed
salt and freshly ground black pepper

FOR THE BURRITOS
4 x 25g/1oz soft tortillas
4 spring onions, trimmed and chopped
25g/1oz reduced fat Cheddar
cheese, grated

TO SERVE
vegetables or a crisp green salad

To make the filling, put the onion, garlic and stock in a heavy-based saucepan and bring to the boil for 5–10 minutes. Reduce the heat, uncover the pan and simmer for 20–30 minutes, until the onion is tender, golden and syrupy.

Add the pepper and chilli and cook for 5 minutes, until softened, then add the tomatoes and chickpeas and simmer for 20 minutes until thickened. Season.

Preheat the oven to 180°C/Gas 4. Put a little of the filling in the centre of each tortilla (you will have some left over). Sprinkle with most of the spring onions, then fold each tortilla around the filling like a parcel, folding in the sides to seal it. Secure with wooden cocktail sticks, if necessary, and arrange in an ovenproof dish.

Pour the remaining filling over the top, then sprinkle with the Cheddar. Bake in the oven for 15 minutes, until hot and bubbling on top. Sprinkled with the remaining spring onions and serve immediately with vegetables or a crisp green salad.

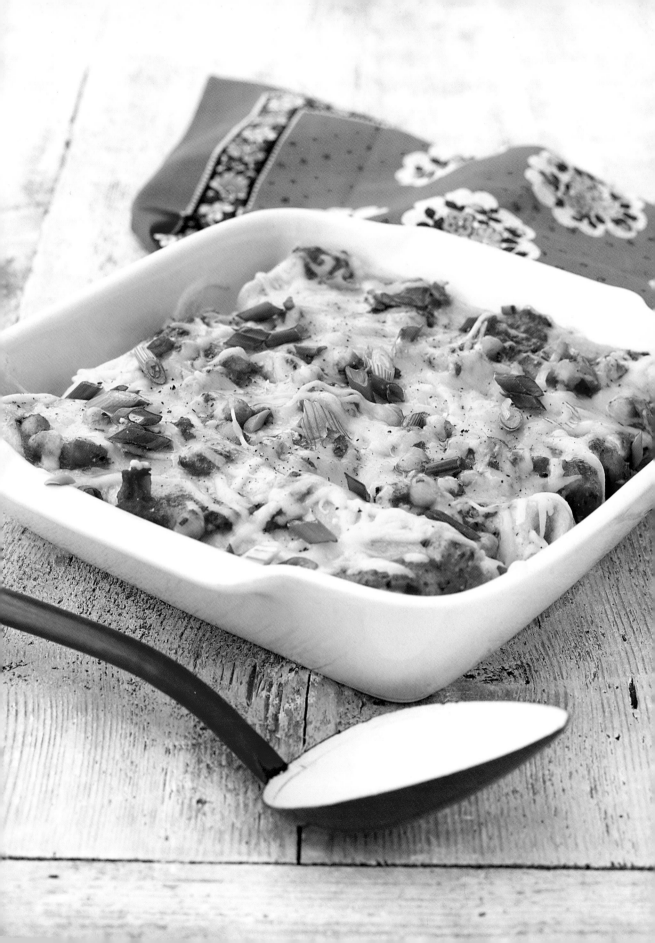

Mexican garbanzos

SERVES 4

WORTH THE EFFORT ❄

Syns per serving
Extra Easy: 1½
Green: 2½
Original: 11

Preparation time 15 minutes
Cooking time 25 minutes

low calorie cooking spray
2 onions, peeled and chopped
2 garlic cloves, peeled and crushed
2 lean back bacon rashers, chopped
1 red pepper, deseeded and chopped
1–2 red chillies, deseeded
and finely chopped
½ tsp dried oregano
450g/1lb tomatoes, chopped
1 tbsp tomato purée
600g/1lb 6oz canned
chickpeas, drained and rinsed
salt and freshly ground black pepper
2 tbsp chopped coriander

TO SERVE
4 tbsp fat free natural fromage frais
1 small red chilli, deseeded
and finely chopped
50g/2oz avocado flesh, diced

There are many different variations on this popular Mexican dish, which is great for breakfast or brunch. The combination of soft chickpeas with spiced tomato sauce works very well. It's delicious served with tortillas (4½ Syns per 25g/1oz), if wished.

Spray a large non-stick frying pan with low calorie cooking spray and place over a medium heat. Add the onions, garlic and bacon and cook for 5 minutes. Add the pepper and chilli and cook for 2–3 minutes, then stir in the oregano, tomatoes, tomato purée and 90ml/3fl oz of water. Bring to the boil, then add the chickpeas and simmer gently for 12–15 minutes. Season and stir in the coriander.

Divide between four plates. Top each serving with some of the fromage frais and sprinkle with the chilli and avocado.

Salmon steaks with fruity salsa

SERVES 4

EASY

Syns per serving
Extra Easy: 1/2
Original: 1/2
Green: 18

Preparation time 15 minutes plus standing
Cooking time 8–10 minutes

1 red onion, peeled and finely chopped
1 small pineapple, peeled and finely chopped
2 oranges, 1 peeled, segmented and chopped and the other juiced
1 small red chilli, deseeded and finely chopped
a small handful of coriander, chopped
salt and freshly ground black pepper
4 x 200g/7oz skinless salmon steaks

The wonderfully fresh and zingy salsa is a fabulous accompaniment to salmon steaks and works equally well served with grilled chicken or prawns.

For the salsa, combine the onion, pineapple, orange segments and juice, chilli and coriander in a small bowl. Season and stand in the fridge for about 1 hour to allow the flavours to combine.

Preheat the grill to medium–hot or prepare the barbecue. Season the salmon steaks then place them under the grill or on the barbecue and cook for 4–5 minutes on each side, or until cooked all the way through. Serve immediately, accompanied with the salsa.

Cajun red snapper

SERVES 4

EASY ✤ (only if fish are fresh)

Syns per serving
Extra Easy: Free
Original: Free
Green: 5

Preparation time 5 minutes
Cooking time 4–6 minutes

FOR THE CAJUN SEASONING
1 tsp cayenne pepper
2 tsp paprika
½ tsp salt
1 tsp garlic powder
1 tsp freshly ground black pepper
½ tsp dried oregano
½ tsp dried thyme

FOR THE RED SNAPPER
4 x 110g/4oz red snapper fillets
low calorie cooking spray

TO SERVE
vegetables or a crisp salad

Most firm-fleshed fish are suitable for this cooking method, which is widely used in the Deep South of the United States. We've chosen red snapper but you could use salmon, sea bass or swordfish.

To make the Cajun seasoning, mix all the ingredients together in a bowl. Spray the red snapper fillets with low calorie cooking spray and dip them into the Cajun seasoning, until they are well coated.

Heat a cast-iron frying pan or grill pan over a high heat until it is really hot (these pans will give the best result but you can use an ordinary frying pan).

Put the coated fillets into the hot pan and cook for 2–3 minutes, until their undersides look blackened and charred. Turn them over and cook the other sides.

Serve immediately with vegetables or a crisp salad.

Chargrilled Tex-Mex prawns with lime and mango salsa

SERVES 4

EASY

Syns per serving
Extra Easy: Free
Original: Free
Green: 5½

Preparation time 10 minutes
Cooking time 4–6 minutes

24 large raw tiger or king prawns, peeled
low calorie cooking spray

FOR THE LIME AND MANGO SALSA
2 ripe mangoes, peeled, stoned and cut into 1cm/½in dice
1 red pepper, deseeded and cut into 1cm/½in dice
110g/4oz pineapple, cut into 1cm/½in dice
juice of 2 limes
a small handful of chopped mint and flat-leaf parsley
salt and freshly ground black pepper

The Tex-Mex flavours and textures of this piquant salsa are a perfect marriage for the chargrilled prawns.

Make the lime and mango salsa by combining all the ingredients together in a bowl and seasoning well. Set aside.

Preheat the grill to medium–hot or heat a griddle. Lightly spray the prawns with low calorie cooking spray and season well. Place under the grill or on the griddle and cook for 2–3 minutes on each side, or until the prawns turn pink and are cooked through.

Divide the prawns between four warmed plates and serve with the salsa.

Louisiana gumbo

SERVES 4

WORTH THE EFFORT ❄ (only if fish are fresh)

Syns per serving
Extra Easy: Free
Original: 4
Green: 5½

Preparation time 15 minutes
Cooking time 1½ hours

2 onions, peeled and chopped
1 green pepper, deseeded and chopped
2 celery sticks, chopped
1 garlic clove, peeled and crushed
1.25 litres/2 pints fish or vegetable stock
½ tsp dried thyme
1 bay leaf
2 tsp paprika
1 tsp cayenne pepper
360ml/12fl oz passata
225g/8oz raw king prawns, peeled
225g/8oz fresh crab meat, boiled
salt and freshly ground black pepper
a dash of Tabasco sauce
4 spring onions, trimmed and thinly sliced

TO SERVE
225g/8oz boiled rice

This spicy dish is very popular in New Orleans, the home of jazz. A gumbo is almost soupy in consistency and is served simply with plain boiled rice.

Put the onions, pepper, celery, garlic and 300ml/½ pint of the stock in a large heavy-based saucepan, cover and bring to the boil. Boil for 5–10 minutes, then uncover and simmer gently for 20–30 minutes, until the onions are tender and syrupy.

Add the thyme, bay leaf, paprika, cayenne pepper, passata and the remaining stock, then leave to simmer for 45 minutes.

Stir in the prawns and crab meat, and season. Cook over a low heat for a further 10 minutes, until the prawns are cooked and have turned pink.

Check the seasoning and adjust if necessary, add the Tabasco sauce and stir in the spring onions. Divide the rice between four deep bowls, top with the gumbo and serve.

Chilli con carne

SERVES 4

EASY ❄

Syns per serving
Extra Easy: Free
Original: 2½
Green: 7½

Preparation time 15 minutes
Cooking time 45 minutes

low calorie cooking spray
1 large onion, peeled
and finely chopped
2 garlic cloves, peeled and crushed
2 red chillies, deseeded and chopped
2 tsp ground cumin
1 tsp ground coriander
1 tsp paprika
a pinch of cayenne pepper
450g/1lb extra lean minced beef
400g can chopped tomatoes
1 tbsp tomato purée
300ml/½ pint beef stock
salt and freshly ground black pepper
200g/7oz canned red kidney beans,
drained and rinsed

TO SERVE
chopped coriander

The name of this dish is an anglicised version of its correct Spanish name, 'chile con carne' meaning 'peppers with meat'. There is a lot of controversy over where the dish originated but the recipe has evolved and there are now many different styles and regional variations – ours is based on a Texan recipe.

Spray a large saucepan with low calorie cooking spray and place over over a low heat. Fry the onion gently for 6–8 minutes, until softened and golden. Add the garlic, chillies and all the spices and continue frying, stirring occasionally, for 2–3 minutes, to release the aroma of the spices.

Add the beef, tomatoes, tomato purée and stock. Stir well and bring to the boil. Reduce the heat, cover and leave to simmer gently for 20–25 minutes, until the liquid is reduced.

Season, add the kidney beans and heat them through gently for about 5 minutes. Sprinkle with chopped coriander and serve hot.

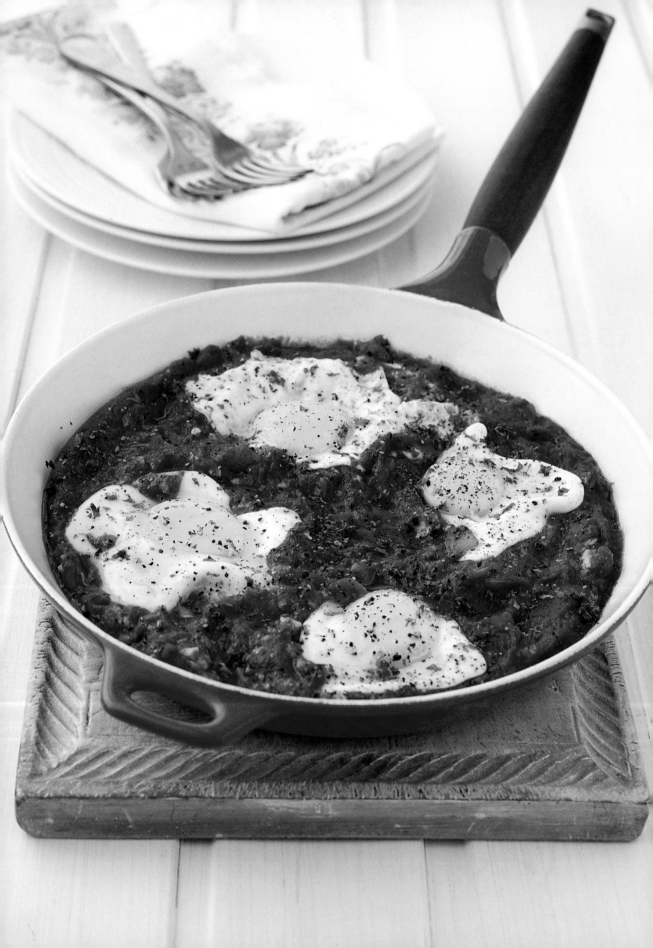

Huevos rancheros

SERVES 4

EASY ⊛

Syns per serving
Extra Easy: Free
Original: Free
Green: 6

Preparation time 20 minutes
Cooking time under 1½ hours

350g/12oz lean bacon lardons
1 onion, peeled and finely chopped
2 garlic cloves, peeled
and finely chopped
1 red chilli, deseeded and finely diced
1 red pepper, deseeded
and finely chopped
2 x 400g cans chopped tomatoes
1 tsp artificial sweetener
1 tsp ground cinnamon
1 tsp ground cumin
4 medium eggs

TO SERVE
chopped coriander
a green salad (optional)

Translated as 'ranch style eggs', this hearty dish with tomatoes and eggs makes for a special breakfast or brunch, or even a light lunch when served with a crisp green salad.

Heat a large non-stick frying pan over a medium heat. Stir in the bacon, onion, garlic, chilli and pepper and cook over a medium heat for 8–10 minutes. Then add the tomatoes, sweetener, cinnamon and cumin and bring to the boil. Reduce the heat and cook for 40–45 minutes or until the mixture is very thick, stirring occasionally.

Preheat the oven to 200°C/Gas 6. Transfer the tomato mixture to a large, shallow ovenproof frying pan or dish. Level the surface and make four shallow, evenly spaced 'hollows' in the mixture with the back of a spoon.

Carefully break an egg into each 'hollow' and place in the oven for 20–25 minutes or until the eggs have set. Remove from the oven, garnish with chopped coriander, and serve with a green salad, if wished.

New York-style meatloaf

SERVES 4

EASY ❋

Syns per serving
Extra Easy: 5
Original: 5
Green: 17½

Preparation time 10 minutes
Cooking time 1¾ hours

500g/1lb 2oz extra lean minced beef
250g/9oz extra lean minced pork
1 red pepper, deseeded and
very finely diced
8 spring onions, trimmed
and finely sliced
4 tbsp finely chopped flat-leaf parsley
1 egg, beaten
1 tsp English mustard
1 garlic clove, peeled and crushed
110g/4oz fresh wholemeal breadcrumbs
salt and freshly ground black pepper
400g can cherry tomatoes, drained

TO SERVE
chopped basil (optional)

You can make this spiced meatloaf up to two days ahead of eating – simply cover and chill in the fridge until you are ready and then re-heat in the oven or serve at room temperature.

Preheat the oven to 180°C/Gas 4. Place all the ingredients, except the cherry tomatoes in a large mixing bowl, seasoning well. Knead the mixture with your hands until well combined.

Line a medium-sized loaf tin with non-stick baking parchment and transfer the mixture to the tin. Bake in the oven for 1½ hours or until cooked through. The meat should shrink away from the sides of the tin when cooked. Remove from the oven and allow to rest for 15–20 minutes, then turn out on to a baking sheet. Place the cherry tomatoes on top and return to the oven for 12–15 minutes. Garnish with basil, if using, carve the loaf into thick slices and serve.

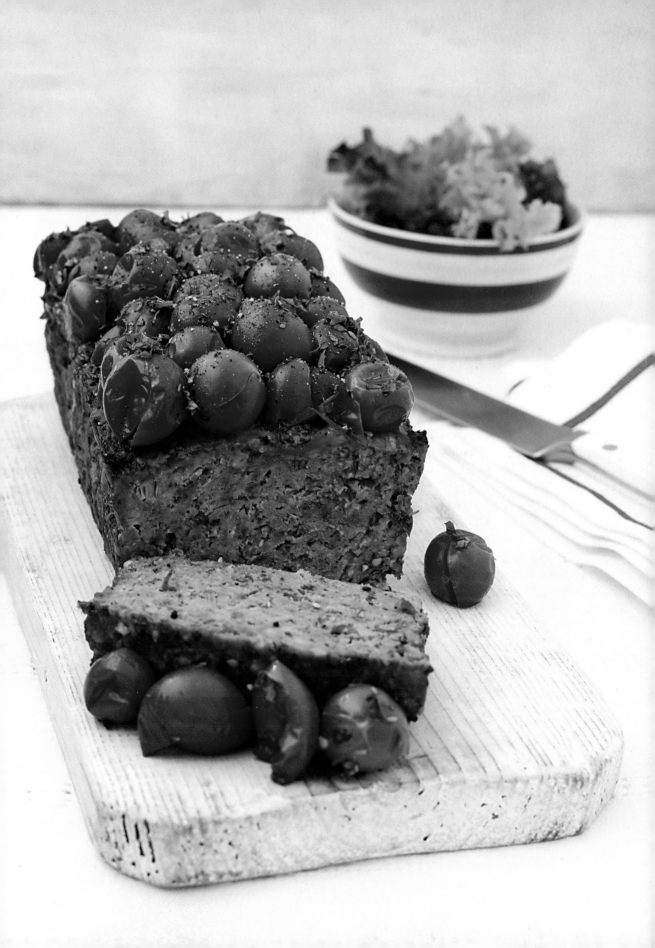

Real McCoy quarter pounders

SERVES 4

EASY

Syns per serving
Extra Easy: ½
Original: ½
Green: 7½

Preparation time 10 minutes
Cooking time 10 minutes

450g/1lb extra lean minced beef
1 small onion, peeled
and finely chopped
1 tbsp tomato ketchup
1 egg, beaten
salt and freshly ground black pepper
low calorie cooking spray

TO SERVE
lettuce leaves
slices of tomato and pickled gherkins
a crisp salad

What could be more American than a real hamburger with all the trimmings? For a healthy, low-fat version of the classic burger, use extra lean minced beef.

Mix the beef in a bowl with the onion, tomato ketchup, egg and seasoning. Divide the mixture into four equal portions and shape into thick patties with your hands.

Preheat the grill to hot or prepare the barbecue. Spray the burgers with low calorie cooking spray and place them on a grill rack under the grill or on the barbecue. Cook for about 5 minutes on each side, depending on how you like them cooked. They should be coloured and slightly charred on the outside and juicy and moist inside.

Serve the hot burgers on a bed of lettuce leaves, acccompanied with sliced tomato, gherkins and a crisp salad.

Spicy buffalo wings with dips

SERVES 4

EASY

Syns per serving
Extra Easy: 2½
Original: 2½
Green: 8

Preparation time 10 minutes plus marinating
Cooking time 25 minutes

FOR THE MARINADE
2 tbsp runny honey
3 tbsp soy sauce
2 garlic cloves, peeled and crushed
1 tsp paprika
1 red chilli, deseeded and finely chopped
1 tsp Tabasco or hot pepper sauce
1 tbsp white wine vinegar
2 tbsp tomato ketchup

FOR THE BUFFALO WINGS
16 skinless chicken wings

FOR THE HONEY MUSTARD DIP
110g/4oz fat free natural fromage frais
2 tsp Dijon mustard
2 tsp runny honey

FOR THE HERBY YOGURT DIP
110g/4oz fat free natural yogurt
a small bunch of chives, chopped
salt

TO SERVE
a crisp salad

These sticky, spicy chicken wings have nothing whatever to do with buffaloes! But they are very popular in the United States and are usually eaten with delicious dips. Here, we've provided recipes for honey mustard and herby yogurt dips.

Mix together all the marinade ingredients in a large bowl, add the chicken wings and turn them around in the marinade until they are completely coated. Cover and leave in a cool place for 30 minutes.

Preheat the oven to 200°C/Gas 6. Put the coated chicken wings on a baking sheet and brush them with any leftover marinade. Cook in the oven for about 25 minutes, until the chicken is cooked and crisp. Brush once or twice with the marinade during cooking.

For the honey mustard dip, mix together the fromage frais, mustard and honey in a small bowl.

For the herby yogurt dip, mix together the yogurt, chives and salt, in another small bowl.

Serve the buffalo wings with the dips and a crisp salad.

Steak pizzaiola

SERVES 4

EASY ❄

Syns per serving
Extra Easy: Free
Original: 6
Green: 13

Preparation time 15 minutes
Cooking time under 25 minutes

1 large onion, peeled
and finely chopped
3 garlic cloves, peeled
and finely chopped
100ml/3½fl oz beef stock
400g can cherry tomatoes
600g/1lb 6oz potatoes, peeled
and cut into 1.5cm/½in dice
low calorie cooking spray
1 tsp dried rosemary
4 x 200g/7oz lean fillet or sirloin steaks
6 tbsp finely chopped oregano
6 tbsp finely chopped flat-leaf parsley
salt and freshly ground black pepper

TO SERVE
green beans

For a change, try using escalopes of chicken or pork instead of steaks (just make sure they are cooked through before serving).

Place a large non-stick frying pan over a medium heat. Add the onion, garlic and stock and cook, stirring, for 5–6 minutes or until soft. Add the tomatoes and simmer gently for 10–12 minutes.

Meanwhile, boil the potatoes in a large saucepan of lightly salted water for 8–10 minutes. Drain thoroughly and spray the saucepan with low calorie cooking spray. Sauté the potatoes over a high heat for 3–4 minutes until golden and tender. Transfer to a bowl, sprinkle with the rosemary and keep warm.

Heat a large, ridged grill pan over a high heat. Add the steaks and cook for 3–5 minutes on each side, until cooked to your liking. Remove from the pan, cover with foil and allow to rest for 5 minutes.

Add the herbs to the tomato mixture and season well. Remove from the heat.

Divide the tomato mixture between four warmed plates and top with the steaks. Serve with the sautéed potatoes and green beans.

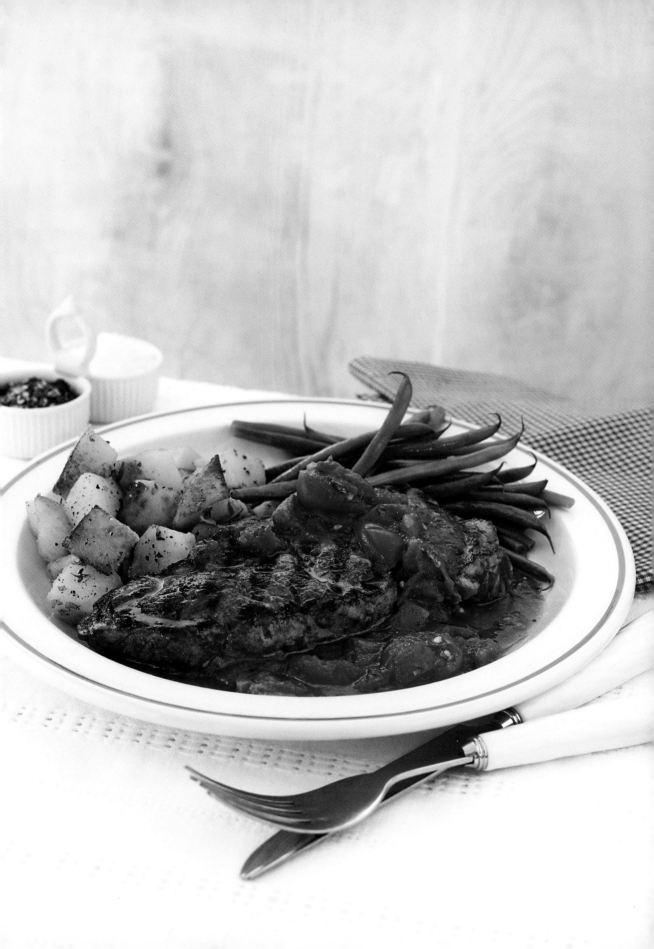

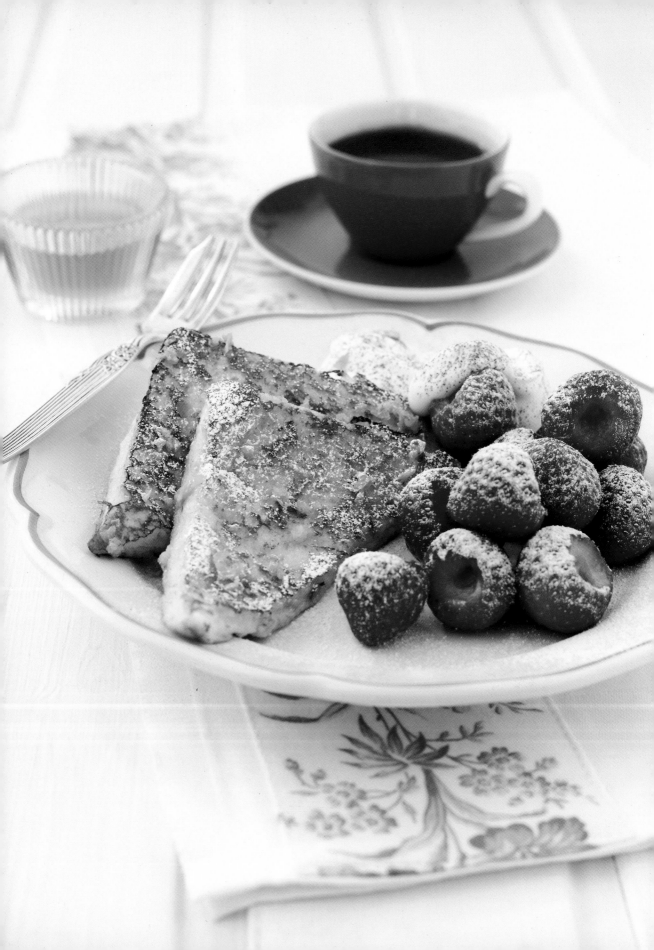

French toast with strawberries

SERVES 4

EASY (V)

Syns per serving
Extra Easy: 4½
Original: 4½
Green: 4½

Preparation time 5 minutes plus soaking
Cooking time 6–8 minutes

2 eggs
150ml/¼ pint skimmed milk
artificial sweetener, to taste
a dash of vanilla extract
1 tsp grated orange zest
4 x 25g/1oz slices white bread
low calorie cooking spray
450g/1lb strawberries

TO SERVE
grated orange zest
1 tsp icing sugar
fat free natural yogurt

In the United States, this would be eaten for breakfast but French toast also makes a delicious dessert. If you like, you can prepare the toast one day ahead, then cover and chill it until you are ready to cook.

In a wide bowl, beat the eggs with the skimmed milk, sweetener, vanilla extract and orange zest.

Dip each slice of bread into the egg mixture and place the slices in a shallow dish. Pour the remaining mixture over the top and set aside for at least 30 minutes.

Spray a large non-stick frying pan with low calorie cooking spray and place over a high heat. Add the bread slices, reduce the heat to low and cook the bread until the slices are golden brown underneath. Flip the slices over and cook the other sides.

Transfer the French toast to four plates and divide the strawberries between them. Garnish with orange zest, dust with the icing sugar and serve each one with a dollop of yogurt.

Key lime pie

SERVES 8

EASY ❄

Syns per serving
Extra Easy: 5½
Original: 5½
Green: 5½

Preparation time 25 minutes
plus chilling
Cooking time 10 minutes

8 reduced fat digestive biscuits,
finely crushed
50g/2oz low fat spread, melted
1 sachet sugar-free lemon
and lime jelly crystals
150ml/¼ pint boiling water
2 tsp powdered gelatine
finely grated zest of 2 limes
juice of 4 limes
a few drops of green food colouring
400g/14oz fat free vanilla yogurt
200g/7oz quark
6–8 tbsp artificial sweetener,
or to taste

FOR THE CANDIED LIMES
2 limes, thinly sliced
6 tbsp artificial sweetener

Flavours of sunny Florida burst through in this simple but tasty dessert that is flavoured with zingy lime juice and zest.

Mix together the biscuits and melted spread and spoon into the base of an 18cm/7in spring-form cake tin. Chill in the fridge for 30 minutes.

Make up the jelly with the boiling water and stir in the gelatine. Leave to cool, then place in a food processor with the lime zest and juice, food colouring, yogurt, quark and sweetener. Blend until smooth and then pour over the biscuit base. Cover and chill in the fridge overnight or until set.

To make the candied limes, cut each lime slice in half and place in a small saucepan with 200ml/7fl oz of water and the sweetener. Bring to the boil, remove from the heat and allow to cool.

To serve, remove the key lime pie from the tin and place on a serving plate. Garnish with the candied limes, cut into wedges and serve.

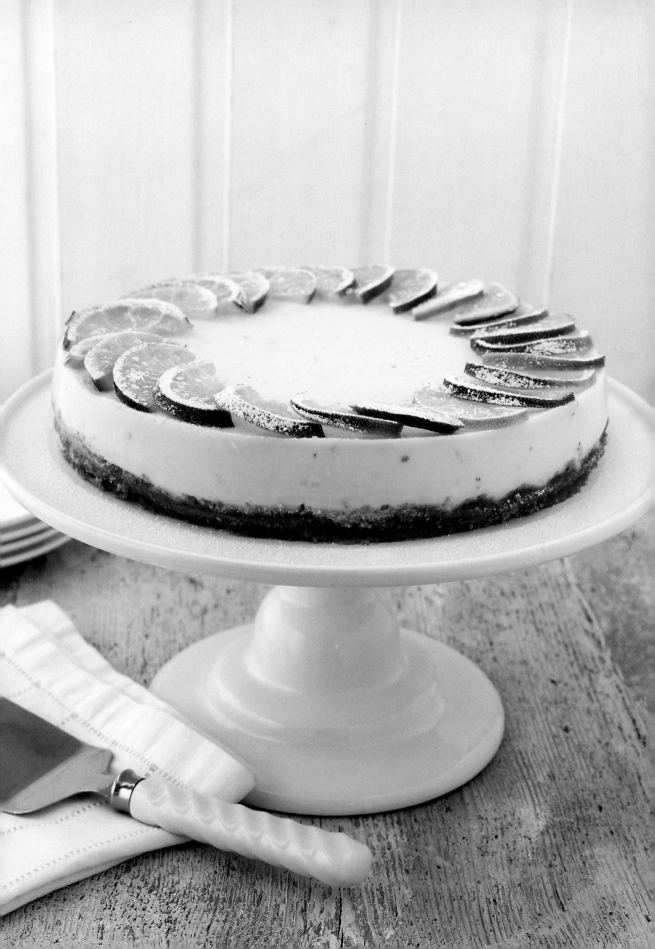

New York-style no-cook cheesecake

SERVES 8

EASY

Syns per serving
Extra Easy: 5
Original: 5
Green: 5

Preparation time 25 minutes
plus chilling

8 reduced fat digestive biscuits,
finely crushed
50g/2oz low fat spread, melted
1 sachet sugar-free
lemon and lime jelly crystals
150ml/¼ pint boiling water
1 tsp powdered gelatine
400g/14oz fat free vanilla yogurt
1–2 tsp vanilla extract
1 tbsp finely grated lemon zest
200g/7oz quark
4–5 tbsp artificial sweetener,
or to taste

TO SERVE
mixed berries of your choice
icing sugar (optional)

The classic New York cheesecake is baked with masses of soft cheese, eggs and cream. Here we have a no-cook, low-Syn dessert that can be made ahead of time.

Mix together the crushed biscuits and melted spread and spoon into the base of a 20cm/8in spring-form cake tin. Chill in the fridge for 30 minutes.

Mix the jelly crystals with the boiling water and stir in the gelatine. Leave to cool, then place in a food processor with the yogurt, vanilla extract, lemon zest, quark and sweetener. Blend until smooth then pour over the biscuit base. Cover and chill in the fridge overnight or until set.

Remove the cheesecake from the tin and place on a serving plate. Arrange mixed berries of your choice over the top and lightly dust with icing sugar (1 Syn per level tsp), if desired. Cut into wedges and serve.

Index

1 3 5 7 9 10 8 6 4 2

Published in 2010 by Ebury Press, an imprint of Ebury Publishing

A Random House Group Company

The Random House Group Limited Reg. No. 954009

Addresses for companies within the Random House Group can be found at www.randomhouse.co.uk

A CIP catalogue record for this book is available from the British Library

The Random House Group Limited supports The Forest Stewardship Council (FSC), the leading international
forest certification organisation. All our titles that are printed on Greenpeace approved FSC certified paper
carry the FSC logo. Our paper procurement policy can be found at www.rbooks.co.uk/environment

To buy books by your favourite authors and register for offers visit www.rbooks.co.uk

Printed and Bound in China by C & C Offset Printing Co., Ltd.

ISBN 9780091933531

Recipes created by Sunil Vijayaker
Design: Two Associates
Recipe photography: Jon Whitaker
Food stylist: Sunil Vijayaker
Prop stylist: Rachel Jukes

FOR SLIMMING WORLD
Founder and chairman: Margaret Miles-Bramwell OBE, FRSA
Managing Director: Caryl Richards
Project Coordinator: Beverley Farnsworth
Text by Christine Michael

PICTURE CREDITS
Inmagine: pages 11, 13, 14
Gareth Morgans: pages 12, 17
iStockphoto: page 18
Bill Morton: page 23
Getty Images: page 25